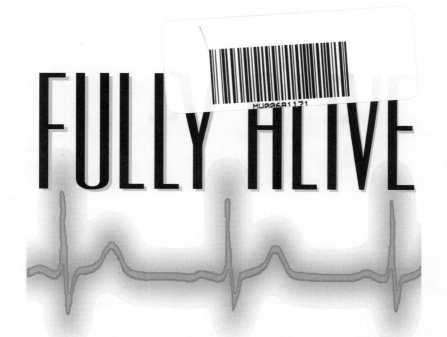

FULLY ALIVE

DISCOVERING

THE ADVENTURE

OF HEALTHY AND

HOLY LIVING

JERRY HULL & LARRY HULL

Beacon Hill Press of Kansas City
Kansas City, Missouri

ISBN 083-411-7266

Printed in the
United States of America

Cover Design: Paul Franitza

Cover Photo: Tony Stone Images / Greg Adams

Library of Congress Cataloging-in-Publication Data

Hull, Jerry D. (Jerry Dean), 1938-
    Fully alive : discovering the adventure of healthy and holy living / Jerry Hull, Larry Hull.
       p.   cm.
    Include bibliographical references.
    ISBN 0-8341-1726-6 (pbk.)
    1. Christian life.   2. Health—Religious aspects—Christianity.
I. Hull, Larry, 1938-
BV4501.2.H8196   1997
248.4—dc21   97-31981
                                               CIP

10 9 8 7 6 5 4 3 2

To
Reeda, Roxie, Barbara, and Karen—
the key women in my life.
Their nearly 200 years of accumulated influence
upon my life has been and continues to be
a source of great affirmation.

JDH

To
Aarlie, L.D., Heather, Amy, Beth, and Dean,
who have added zest, joy, and abundance
to my "Fully Alive" days.

LDH

Contents

INVITATION

JOIN US FOR AN ADVENTURE

We began as a single fertilized egg and, within hours following conception, split and formed separate selves. We attached to the uterus wall within our mother and hung on for dear life. Nine months later, much to Mother's surprise, she delivered twins. We were born during the worst spring blizzard the old-timers in west Texas could remember. For us, that abundant snow has been symbolic of lives blessed with spiritual adventure and shared discoveries.

We are identical twin brothers on a journey of *wholeness*. We are discovering that wholeness is a dynamic, intentional journey of meaning, satisfaction, and faith in God that unfolds each new day. This journey of wholeness moves toward joyous harmony, soul-satisfying integration, and God-pleasing balance as persons. Wholeness engages every part of us—body, mind, soul, and spirit. We share our journey with you in humility, because we know that wholeness as a way of living exceeds our capacity to fully comprehend it. Come travel with us on this road to wholeness. It's the adventure of a lifetime.

—*Jerry Hull*
Larry Hull

INTRODUCTION

AN UNFOLDING VISTA

My son, Tim, and I endure miles of rough and dusty roads on our way to Trinity Lakes. Any summer is incomplete until we journey to this place of renewal and perspective. The excursion is capped by climbing the peaks above the lakes. Here we recognize the majesty of the universe, sense the miracle of life, and understand afresh that a God of compassion, power, and purpose is above us and among us. Tim and I alternate between excited chatter and cautious silence as each new vista of beauty unfolds before us.

Our annual Trinity Lakes outing reminds me of wholeness—a present achievement and a lifelong journey. We find fulfillment in the present moments but recognize our limitations. Like mountain hikers, we realize there are new breathtaking views as we move onward. And just knowing there is more to discover drives us onward.

I learned about wholeness in my kindergarten art class:

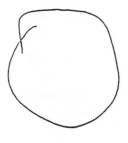 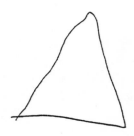 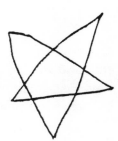

The circle, the triangle, and the star help us grasp the meaning of wholeness. The circle depicts *integration* (building one's life around a single purpose or unified focus), *harmony* (living one's life with inner tranquility and in proper relationship to the Creator and the creation), and *balance* (exhibiting steadiness and stability in all arenas of our life).

INTEGRATION

People who are spiritually, physically, emotionally, and mentally healthy exhibit unity, focus, and consistency. They are not capricious or unpredictable. They order life within a strong core of unshakable values and commitments and a true sense of identity. They pursue activities that are in keeping with who they are.

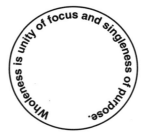

If we want to see what a person looks like, we can look at a photograph. My photograph reveals a bespectacled middle-aged man with a large nose and thin, graying hair. These external features, however, do not reveal who I really am. By grace and confession I am a man in relationship with Christ. The whole of my life is integrated into this focus. The single purpose of my life is to be conformed to the image of Jesus.

HARMONY

People of wholeness are in harmony with the Creator, the created (others), and the creation. They have healthy relationships with the supreme God, the other children of God, and the world around them. Each of us is accountable to maintain harmony in these areas.

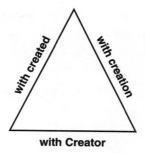

with Creator

BALANCE

People of wholeness tend faithfully to the development of the total person. They work consistently and faithfully to keep their mind, body, spirit, soul (emotions), and social relationships healthy. A star is a single unified figure comprised of five interlocking points. All five points must be present, or the figure is something less than a star. Similarly, if one dimension of our personhood is poorly developed, the potential beauty, strength, and symmetry of our lives is distorted.

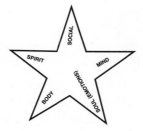

Five parts of a single whole:

I am one part body. I am a physical being. I am bones, blood, and sometimes bunions.

I am one part mind. I am a person of intellectual capacity and curiosity. I have the ability to think, reason, analyze, memorize, and forget.

I am one part spirit. I am a spiritual being. I connect with God, in whose image I have been created. I may communicate with God and participate in His purposes for the world.

I am one part soul. I am an emotional being. I experience feelings and states of consciousness, make volitional choices, and know passions and desires.

I am one part sociocultural. I am a social being. As a social being, I
  interact with others within the context of a particular culture, history, and unique family setting.
I am all five dimensions simultaneously.

We can begin to grasp something of the breadth and depth of
wholeness when we superimpose the triangle, the circle, and the star.

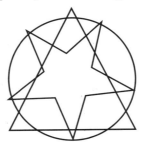

Each of the dimensions illustrated in the three designs factors into the journey of wholeness. My father used to say that if we wanted
to achieve worthy goals or make our dreams come true, it would take
"a heap of livin'." Genuine wholeness is a challenge that requires our
best. We can do it, but not without help.

In this book we claim that wholeness becomes attainable when
we are anchored in Jesus Christ. Our destiny, according to Scripture, is
"to be conformed to the likeness of his Son" (Rom. 8:29). In Christ we
discover what Gal. 5:22-23 calls the "fruit of the Spirit": the inner
graces of "love," "joy," and "peace"; the other related graces of "patience," "kindness," and "goodness"; and the character qualities of
"faithfulness," "gentleness," and "self-control."

Wholeness in Christ is not reserved only for the major-league
players—Mother Teresa, Billy Graham, or Henri Nouwen. Wholeness,
a balanced, holy lifestyle, is being lived out by ordinary folks all over
the world. How fortunate we are when our lives intersect with a real,
live person of wholeness! May it be so for us. May we inspire each
other to become persons of integration, harmony, and balance.

*May God himself, the God who makes everything holy
and whole, make you holy and whole, put you together
—spirit, soul, and body—and keep you fit for the coming of our Master, Jesus Christ. The One who called
you is completely dependable. If he said it, he'll do it!*

—1 Thess. 5:23-24, TM

CHAPTER 1

A WORD FROM THE PROFESSOR . . .
WHOLENESS

Writer Lurette Kerr unmasked the everyday ways we perceive
wholeness. In an article titled "Good Grief, Where Are the Perfect People?" which appeared in the January 1994 issue of *Diabetes Forecast*, she wrote, "When I was diagnosed with Type I diabetes
at age 18, I became suddenly, keenly aware of having joined the ranks
of the 'handicapped,' the 'limited,' the 'flawed.' Driving home from
the doctor's office, my mother advised me to keep 'our secret,' for my
condition would cost me friends, suitors and jobs."

Often we fall into the trap of erroneously believing there are reasons
why we should not anticipate a life of wholeness—at least not now or here
or under these conditions. From painful experience Kerr writes, "Wholeness is not a divine gift bestowed upon a lucky few; it is, rather, something
achieved by those who choose to face life's challenges headon.

"We earn wholeness when we see life's obstacles not as walls,
but as hurdles. With each hurdle that we jump, we come that much
closer to fully realizing our true potential" (ibid.).

We, like Kerr, may look around us or at the mirror that stares
back at us and find limited, flawed, and handicapped people. The

15

journey of wholeness starts with owning our limitations and accepting them as opportunities, challenges, and adventures. This book is for the flawed, limited, handicapped, and injured. That's all of us.

THE LAW OF THE RESERVOIR

Barb and I sometimes escape to a mountain cabin near Anderson Ranch Dam. The view of the reservoir is one of my favorite Idaho scenes. We see the Sawtooth Mountains off in the distance, closer hills rising up from the canyon floor, and a rich blue sky forming a background. The picture for me, however, is not finished until I see the water level in the dam. Nothing quite compares with this scene *if the reservoir is full.*

A full reservoir guarantees life, bountiful life. Full is better than empty. Grouse Creek runs below our mountain cabin and about 300 yards farther flows into the Boise River and on to Anderson Ranch Dam. During eight years of drought that began in the late 1980s, Grouse Creek served as a constant reminder of empty places and situations. Some hot days of midsummer, the creek went completely dry. This past summer, however, the story was different. Even during the hottest and longest days of the summer, Grouse Creek pumped thousands of gallons of water toward the Boise River. The strong gurgling announced that the reservoir would be full—also harvest trucks and Thanksgiving tables.

God is the Source of our fullness. Someone has suggested, "There is a God-shaped hole within each of us." We will never experience fullness until we invite God to fill us with himself.

Throughout this book we plead for choices, actions, and disciplines that lead to personal wholeness. Wholeness describes a person in a healthy alignment/relationship with oneself, with the Creator, with the created (others), and with creation. In addition, a person of wholeness has balance—he or she gives appropriate attention to the multiple dimensions of human existence. A person of wholeness chooses to develop mind, body, soul, and spirit.

Wholeness is both a gift from God and a choice we make. It is God sharing the blessings of himself with us. But to be meaningful, wholeness, like any gift, must be accepted and used. We must make choices and engage in actions that lead from where we are to where we want to be. Our focus is on the present and the future without ignoring the past. We seize today and all our tomorrows as opportunities for growth.

We pursue and are pursued. With every ounce of energy, we seek God. At the same time, He seeks us with a never-ending love. The Incarnation (God coming to earth as Jesus the Son) proves that God wants to be with and among men, women, girls, and boys.

A little Sunday School scholar used bad grammar to state a sublime truth about wholeness. "Jesus Christ is the best picture God ever had took," he said.

We know what God is like by looking at Jesus. God, as Jesus, moved into the neighborhood of humanity. In Bethlehem's barn the fullness of God came among us.

John describes the magnitude of the Incarnation event, God moving in as one of us: "The Word became flesh and made his dwelling among us. We have seen his glory, the glory of the One and Only, who came from the Father, full of grace and truth" (John 1:14). What a wonderful picture God "had took"!

The news gets better—*We can receive Jesus, the fullness of God, into our lives.* Paul wrote, "For in Christ all the fullness of the Deity lives in bodily form, and you have been given fullness in Christ" (Col. 2:9-10). In a letter to the Christians at Ephesus, Paul cites this same theme in the form of a prayer. He prays "that you may be filled to the measure of all the fullness of God" (Eph. 3:19). A bit later in the same letter, Paul repeats the idea of being filled with the fullness of God. He notes that various gifts of ministry are given so that persons in Christ may "attain the whole measure of the fullness of Christ" (Eph. 4:13, author's paraphrase). That's wholeness.

Most of us can say that our lives are full, all right, but of what? Constantly we hear people describe their lives—consumed with work, family, hobbies, meetings, sporting events, and other obligations. Our lives are full, but are we filled with the fullness of God? Consider the experience of chemistry professor Wally Johnson. Johnson wrote these words in his journal:

> Each person has a "carrying capacity" for God. The size is limited only by how empty of other things we are willing to be. . . . There was a crisis moment in my life when I was sick of playing the religious game. In a moment of absolute truth I cried out to God and asked Him to fill me completely.
>
> God's answer was awesome: "I cannot fill you." My response was "God, you can do anything." God replied, "Look at your life. You are full." I was. There was no room or time for God.

By the help of the Holy Spirit I began to remove the "good" of this world so I could be full of the "best" God had for me. I was full of work, tennis, golf, skiing, hunting, fishing, and even jobs [not ministries] in the church.

What Wally discovered at the end of the 20th century, Richard Baxter spoke of in the mid-17th century. In chapter 13 of *The Saints' Everlasting Rest,* he wrote:

Get thy heart as clear from the world as thou canst. Wholly lay by the thoughts of business, troubles, enjoyments, and every thing that may take up any room in thy soul. Get it as empty as thou possibly canst, that it may be more capable of being filled with God. . . .

Thou wilt find as much of God and glory as thy narrow heart is able to contain, and almost nothing to hinder thy full possession but the incapacity of thy own spirit. Then thou wilt think, "O that this understanding and these affections could contain more."

Pastor Daniel Ketchum speaks of "our little kingdom of thingdom." He challenges his parishioners to seek the genuine and authentic goal of life—to know Christ. "Is it Christ plus something that satisfies?" he probes. "Or do we find Christ alone as our source of satisfaction and meaning?"

We may seek wholeness through God's fullness. We may yield every dimension of our lives so that every day in every way we are seeking after God. Each of us may say, "Today I seek all of God to indwell all of me. Tomorrow, as I understand more about myself and God, I will seek a new filling of God's fullness."

Each day I recite a portion of this prayer attributed to St. Patrick:
Christ in the heart of everyone who thinks of me.
Christ in the mouth of everyone who speaks of me.
Christ in every eye that sees me.
Christ in every ear that hears me.

Let's seek the fullness of God and choose wholeness in the dynamics of each new day!

I view happiness as deeper than a momentary good mood—as an enduring sense of positive well-being, an ongoing perception that life is fulfilling, meaningful and pleasant. But in reporting on the markings of happy lives, I define happiness as whatever people mean when they describe their lives as happy rather than unhappy.

—David Myers, *The Pursuit of Happiness*

CHAPTER 2

A WORD FROM THE DOCTOR . . .
HAPPINESS

I am not a philosopher or an expert on happiness. However, I am a happy person. I have learned about happiness from my childhood, my medical practice, my family. For me, happiness is a feeling of inner contentment, of hope and purpose—a lot like being fully alive.

THE SUMMER OF '48

I will never forget the summer of 1948. We lived on the desert plateau of Ontario Heights in eastern Oregon, overlooking the mouth of the Malheur River as it enters the Snake River.

Green was pasted like postage stamps on the brown desert by irrigation canals and ditches watering the thirsty soil. The water poured life into our fields: lush pastures, thigh-high alfalfa, and corn that towered beyond my reach. But coming from this water (or so it was surmised) was bulbar polio myelitis. Children were not allowed to swim in canals and ditches for fear they would contract the deadly, crippling disease. There was an ominous, oppressive fear in our community that summer, a devilish randomness of disease and death that appeared to be lurking behind some hidden shield or force. Who would be next?

In the midst of this uncertainty, our family found joy. My courageous mother was voluntarily caring for people in the polio wards of our local hospital. Pride in our mother and fear of disease wrapped around our lives like the iron lungs encasing the sick ones she served. Dad, who already worked from dawn to dusk, took on many of her chores. My sister Roxie cooked, cleaned, and ran the household; Jerry and I picked up routine but important tasks that Dad could not complete.

From that summer came the grist for many lessons on wholeness:

◆ People who are absorbed in challenging tasks tend to be happy.

That summer, our dairy farm required the collective best that all of us could give. Subtracting Mother's work from the equation exaggerated our own workload and yet magnified our sense of personal importance and worth. The farm wouldn't operate and Mother couldn't volunteer if we didn't all do our part. In the late evening, when Mother's white Plymouth would come down the dusty road and turn into the driveway, we celebrated. We were tired and hot, relieved that our mother was home safe and sound. We knew that she had risked her own health to serve others. And we believed we had contributed to her important mission by doing extra work at home. In the presence of need, our family was not inert and passive. Our prayers and focus were on others. We were involved.

◆ People with a sense of purpose are happy.

Our 1948 family purpose was to share, in a personal way, the tragedies and heartaches of our friends and neighbors. Polio was a contagious disease. The fear that possessed our community that summer was palpable. Who would get it next? And from where? How was it being spread? We believed our mother's kindness and courage made her a hero. As a result, we invested ourselves into a task bigger and beyond each or all of us. We had a common cause.

◆ People with healthy, supportive relationships are happy.

Because large and unnecessary gatherings were discouraged to avoid the spread of polio, our family became especially close that summer. We pulled together as never before, appreciating our health, our friendships, and each other.

The physician was born in me that summer. I sensed that I wanted to be involved in issues of life and death. Mother's example and support were an important influence on my destiny.

CASE HISTORIES

Let me tell you about two patients. I'll summarize their medical charts:

Patient 1: Mrs. Moore is a 78-year-old, homebound female who experienced an acute onset of low back pain while moving from bed to wheelchair. Over the past six to eight months, she has noted progressive weakness. She has lost the functional skills to care for herself. In-house help is necessary 24 hours a day.

Diagnosis: Chronic progressive osteoporosis, with acute lumbar vertebrae compression fracture

Personal note: Mrs. Moore and I had a lovely chat today. In the process, she learned that today was my son's birthday. She asked about him. I told her about a concern I had for him. She prayed. It was a personal prayer for me and my son.

Follow-up: Mrs. Moore advised me that she continues to pray for me and my son. She prayed for us today. She has amazing vitality for life despite her deteriorating health.

Patient 2: Mr. Adams stumbled while at work. He sustained a blow to the great toe. Swelling and pain have persisted.

Diagnosis: Fractured toe

Personal note: July 1991 through October 1991—Mr. Adams is suffering with persistent pain. He states he cannot work because of severe pain in his foot. He wants pain medications and desires more time off from work.

Follow-up: Mr. Adams is still not back to work. He is seeking a disability settlement and appears depressed.

There is a disturbing contrast between Mrs. Moore and Mr. Adams.

Mrs. Moore had a severe physical disease with advanced disability but was gloriously alive, vibrant, and happy. Mr. Adams had a minor toe injury and a trainload of problems. He was in a "poor me" mode: "I can't work. It's not my fault. Someone please compensate me."

Each time I visited Mrs. Moore, I would burst into her hospital room with an expectant spirit. I knew I would be richer, better, lifted, and warmed because of the joy she exuded. To be sure, we talked about physical pain, neuromuscular weakness, soft and fragile bones, and the latest advances in the treatment of osteoporosis. I adjusted her physical therapy, renewed medications, and outlined appropriate strategies for the next couple of months. Mostly we talked about the good things happening in our lives.

In contrast, when Mr. Adams would come to my office, I would reach for his chart, see the name, go through the process of retrieving his history from my memory file, and say to myself, "Oh, no!" Then I would pray for wisdom and strength to be a great orthopedist for a needy person. Most of my orthopedic patients heal, move on, and return to their previous life circumstances, and I feel privileged to have dressed the wounds while God healed them. But with Mr. Adams, I would bolster myself by remembering Mother Teresa's prayer: "I can love only one person at a time. I can pick up only one person at a time. I can feed only one person at a time."

So knowing that Mr. Adams was my "one person" at that time, I would step into the exam room with a smile on my face, my hand outstretched, and my ears open to listen.

Despite reviewing the history, physically examining him, studying the X rays, and recommending treatment, there was never a moment of closure. There was no apparent relief to his suffering. He came to my office unhappy. He left unhappy. Even though I had examined, admonished, encouraged, treated, and advised him, my orthopedic care could not relieve his unhappiness.

We can learn some valuable lessons from Mrs. Moore and Mr. Adams:

◆ Happiness is most often a choice.

Mrs. Moore had decided that her physical circumstances would not dictate the course of her life and the happiness she would experience. Being happy was a choice she made each morning when she woke. Instead of focusing on negative circumstances, she concentrated her thoughts and actions on the many positive moments and people in her life.

Each one of us makes a choice each day: we dwell on our ills, or we search for ways to bring light to the shadows, hope to the discouraged, and cheer to the disheartened. If we choose wisely, we will experience the very things we try to give.

◆ People who care for their souls are happy.

Happiness is clearly created by God. It is woven into the very fabric of life. Happiness is always and abundantly available to the soul that seeks it.

Mrs. Moore had a body full of pain but a happy soul. Her hope and her faith were in God.

Mr. Adams, on the other hand, experienced as much unhappiness as Mrs. Moore experienced happiness, even though his body was much better off than hers.

In 1963 I was a capable, success-oriented medical student at the University of Washington. But I was struggling with issues of faith and temptation in my life. One Sunday after an inspiring worship service, I prayed that my faith in the Living God would be real, current, and powerful and provide me with inner purity and peace. I experienced an amazing, radical change in my thinking, in my direction, and consequently in my entire life. I realized that God knew me individually and that nothing could ever separate me from His love. That day, I fully comprehended that I was a created being. I was not an accident in a meaningless, purposeless, cosmic explosion. I understood that God invented matter, that He invested His great creative self in the world and specifically in the design of our bodies. And though I would continue to be a part of the world of reason, I could not ignore the world of faith.

Infinitesimal Pleasures

The happiness of life is made of minute fractions—the little common, soon forgotten charities of a kiss or smile, a kind look, a heartfelt compliment—countless infinitesimals of pleasurable and genial feelings.
—Samuel Taylor Coleridge

I am happy this week. A few notes from my journal will tell you why.

Friday, August 9. Shot baskets with my son, Dean. He is very good.
. . . My wife, Aarlie, and I had dinner with our children, Beth and
Dean—wonderful kids. Beth is excited about leaving for college. I pray
she will have a godly roommate.

Saturday, August 10. I went on a four-mile jog tonight. It was an
exhilarating run to the church on a cool evening.

Sunday, August 11. Today's church services were great. I was in-
spired by the testimonies of three different people whose lives have been
changed by faith in the Living God.

You see, we can learn a lot about happiness from our families
and friends.

◆ Happiness is about living.

You will discover it in the everyday moments of your life. Excerpts
from my diary document nothing dramatic, great, or world changing—
just a series of small, meaningful, happy events connected together, hand
in hand by the people whom I love and who are part of my life.

◆ Happiness thrives in simplicity.

Early in my marriage I was in the military, stationed in Salt Lake
City on a short-term assignment. Aarlie and I had an infant child. We
had no family nearby. I had no hospital assignments. We did not own a
home. We were not members of any clubs or organizations. Our lives
consisted of caring for each other, working simple eight-hour day jobs,
and attending a small church filled with loving people. We didn't worry about investments, retirement, business success, employees, position, or prestige. This was an uncomplicated, happy time in our lives.

Since then, our lives have become steadily more complex. Four
more children, a house, writing deadlines, a large medical practice, and
all the accompaniments have put us on a faster track, and the journey is
not so simple anymore. Sometimes I have to consciously choose simplicity. I have to remind myself that I personally do not make the world go
around. My delusions of grandeur are just that, delusions.

◆ Happiness is a universal feeling.

Whether it's Salt Lake City or Santo Domingo, Dominican Re-
public, happiness is the same. The potential for happiness knows no

geographical, financial, or social limits. I have met happy people on my mission trips to third world countries. I know many happy people in my own neighborhood.

◆ Happiness is now, not later.

Our time in Salt Lake City helped me see the danger of the "someday syndrome": "Someday we'll have our own home." "Someday we'll have more money." "Someday we'll be close to our families." Someday . . . someday . . . someday . . . ad infinitum. Happiness can be grasped only one moment at a time: a flower, a kind word, a warm sweater, a friend, a soft breeze. Happiness sometimes surprises us in an unexpected evening out, a canceled appointment, or an unplanned delay. Happiness cannot be hoarded or saved; it can only be experienced.

> **No matter what looms ahead, if you can eat today, enjoy the sunlight today, mix good cheer with friends today, enjoy and bless God for it. Do not look back on happiness—or dream of it in the future. You're only sure about today; do not let yourself be cheated out of it.**
>
> —Henry Ward Beecher

The "now" quality of happiness is evident to me as our children grow, mature, and leave our home to make their own. The happinesses we experienced in the past are memories that bring happiness now.

◆ Happiness comes as we give up our expectations.

We are never as important as we dreamed we would be. We don't make as much money or have the power we thought we would.

I am not the surgeon general of the United States. I am a long way from being rich, and sometimes I don't have enough power to control my own day.

> **Happiness is, in part, related to the ratio between expectations and achievements.**
>
> —William James

It is true that we can control many aspects of our lives. Our choices often play a major role in the good and bad things that happen to us. Having a sense of mastery over our lives contributes significantly to our overall sense of well-being. But there are times when things are not going our way. We're down on our luck. It's a bad day, maybe a bad week, maybe even a bad year. That may be a time when we need to give up some of our expectations.

For me, happiness has included accepting the "death of dreams." I call these *course corrections*. I've had to make course corrections in all areas of my life—personal, family, church, and professional.

My children were excellent runners in high school. Watching them run track, set records, and receive recognition for their successes was a real thrill for me.

But two of my "track star" children decided they didn't want to compete anymore and chose to pursue other interests. It was hard for me to make a course correction. I had to give up an expectation. Once I did we were all happier.

◆ Happiness requires taking time for fun.

Experts agree that a little goofing off goes a long way. You don't need to set aside hours to reap the benefits. Try building little blocks of fun into your day. Angela Ebron gives some suggestions in a February 1, 1996, *Family Circle* article: Join in with the kids when they're playing tag, or take a ride on your son's skateboard when you find it in the driveway. Sure, you may feel silly when your backside meets the ground, but you'll also have a good laugh, and a hearty guffaw can do wonders for you. *Think of goofing off as productive; think of it as a minivacation.* It releases tension and soothes and renews you. It causes your whole body to get into a state of deep relaxation.

Great ways to relax:

1. Work up a sweat once in a while. Aerobic activity is known to reduce tension.
2. Carve out little breaks into your schedule. Have moments of relaxation.
3. Pad your schedule. It always seems to take longer to do things than what you planned, and padding your schedule will help remove some of the pressure from deadlines.

4. Kill the ump. Well, don't actually. But find someway to blow off steam such as attending sports events, playing a tough game of racquetball, chopping wood.
5. Soak in a hot tub. Many studies show that a restful hot bath is very relaxing.
6. Get a grip. Keep a hand exerciser or tennis ball in your desk. Just squeezing it in repetitive motions will give you a moment of relaxation.
7. Live longer—be a volunteer. Isolation can magnify your worries. Helping other people will give you a sense of accomplishment and self-respect.
8. Trade in your Jag for a Hyundai. Living above your means can actually make you sick and add a lot of unnecessary stress to your life.
9. Carry a humor first-aid kit. Recently we took a vacation, and our kids brought along a joke book about Norwegians. We laughed for most of the trip. (My wife is Scandinavian.)
10. Smell an apple. Pick some flowers. Pleasant smells tend to be very relaxing.
11. Quit the bowling league. Are you doing too much? If you never have a weeknight free, you're too busy.

I am fascinated by genetic engineering. The DNA of each cell of my body is exactly the same—yet unique to me (well, in my case, unique to me and Jerry).

As our understanding of DNA expands, we are learning more about genetics and the way our DNA affects our bodies and personalities. Genetic engineering can change everything from a tomato plant's resistance against rot to disease processes in animals and humans. Changing the DNA of a cell can be done by inserting into the cell a common virus carrying a different piece of protein.

If something as "simple" as a virus can change us, consider how powerful our own attitudes, emotions, and minds must be on the working of each cell. Even more incredible is the power of God to enter each cell of our body and do the divine genetic engineering needed in order for us to become a different person. It can happen. God can do it. We are not trapped. We can be changed. We can be happier. We can experience the miracle of a new beginning.

Your body is a temple of the Holy Spirit, who is in you *(1 Cor. 6:19)*.

Therefore, if anyone is in Christ, he is a new creation; the old has gone, the new has come! *(2 Cor. 5:17)*.

I have told you this so that my joy may be in you and that your joy may be complete *(John 15:11)*.

DOCTOR'S ORDERS: RX FOR HAPPINESS

1. Work daily on the superficial, temporary, but important aspects of happiness:

   ▶ Choose realistic goals and expectations.

   ▶ Choose to be happy, positive, and enthusiastic.

   ▶ Practice simplicity.

   ▶ Involve yourself in meaningful tasks and work.

   ▶ Avoid the "someday syndrome."

2. Spend a lifetime pursuing the deep and long-term solutions for wholeness that result in happiness.

   ▶ Form open, sincere, and supportive relationships with friends and family.

   ▶ Nurture your soul.

   ▶ Develop a life purpose and a sense of self-realization.

   ▶ Actively seek to know God.

The pain of loss, the pain of illness, the pain of depression, the emotional pain that comes from so many unfilled needs, the pain of worry about loved ones, particularly children and their troubles, these kinds of pains are not due to commitment to God, but are just part of life. The comforting phenomenon, however, is the fact that they can all be incorporated into our life with God and can facilitate an even greater intimacy with Jesus, because it allows us to share with Him all these hurts and anxieties, and find in His friendship the comfort and guidance we need.

—Joseph P. Girzone in *Never Alone*

CHAPTER 3

A WORD FROM THE DOCTOR . . .
PAIN

Pain, suffering, and loss are significant and unavoidable dimensions of everyone's life. Frequently our troubles are of our own making. Sometimes they are just part of ordinary living. C. S. Lewis in *The Problem of Pain* advises, "Try to exclude the possibility of suffering which the order of nature and the existence of free wills involve, and you find that you have excluded life itself." Martin Luther King Jr. agreed. "What does not destroy me makes me stronger," he said.

Most physical pain begins when a raw nerve ending is stimulated and sends a message through a series of nerve pathways to the brain: "Get your hand off that hot stove." "Lift your foot off that sharp glass."

The brain must then figure out what to do: fight or flee, respond or ignore, adapt or accept. It is in this sorting out of stimulus and response that the mental aspect of pain becomes apparent. Physical *suffering* is something that happens in the conscious, interpretative, subjective level of the mind. Suffering takes pain; it is rooted in pain—but it becomes something more.

Dr. Mitchell J. Cohen writes, "As pain becomes chronic, it begins to dominate our mental life. All activities are seen through the lens of chronic pain, and many activities may be avoided due to the fear of pain. Pain then seems to be properly called SUFFERING. The suffering starts to control you and me instead of us adapting or changing or moving away from the noxious stimulus."

CHRONIC PAIN CAN HURT

The old saying that "pain can't kill you" is a myth. Chronic pain can destroy even the strongest person.

Chronic pain is dangerous to us as a total organism because it results in

◆ *Decreased activity.* This leads to a sedentary lifestyle and a greater risk of coronary heart disease, weight gain, and hypertension, plus loss of agility, strength, and lung expansion.

◆ *Decreased immune function.* Chronic pain can decrease the ability of the immune system to function at maximum performance, thereby increasing the risk of infection, cancer, and other opportunistic diseases.

◆ *Depression and associated mental disturbances.*

The stoic approach to pain—"Grit your teeth and bear it"—has its time and place but is not an option for the chronic sufferer.

MILE 22

I ran my first marathon in Victoria, British Columbia, in the fall of 1988. I was confident that I was prepared. As part of my training, I had run up to 20 miles on several occasions. The day was cool and overcast, but the atmosphere was festive. My family had come to help me celebrate this colossal event in my life.

There were about 5,000 runners, and the race was progressing wonderfully. At mile 14, 15, and 18 my wife, Aarlie, and the kids found me. They drove by slowly, aiming cameras at me and cheering loudly. Mile 20 was my last contact with them. They headed to the finish line to cheer me in. I was running easily, faster by about 15 seconds per mile than I had planned. I expected to finish at about 3 hours and 45 minutes. Not bad for a 48-year-old runner with a foot drop on his first marathon!

At mile 22 I hit "the wall." This is the point at which you've come to the end of your "hoarded resources" of muscle glucose (sugar) and you begin to burn body fat. From a nonscientific standpoint—you're exhausted! I found myself going slower and slower, and finally ended up walking with an occasional jog for short distances. The curbs seemed almost impossible to climb. The slightest incline felt as if it would destroy me. I wanted to quit, and if I could have saved face, I would have. I was in pain. I was suffering mentally, physically, and emotionally.

At the finish line Aarlie was getting worried. I was well over my anticipated time of 3 hours and 45 minutes She heard a siren and saw an ambulance head back along the course. She was sure they were going for me. However, with persistence, determination, and much pain and suffering, I managed to make it across the finish line in 3 hours and 54 minutes.

I fell into the arms of Aarlie and my daughters, Heather and Amy. They helped me to an open area, and I collapsed on the grass. They lifted and massaged my legs and gave me fluids and fruit. After about 20 to 30 minutes, with my arms draped over their shoulders, I was finally able to make it the few blocks to the van. I crawled into the back and stayed there for the next several hours.

By the following day I could barely walk, let alone negotiate the stairs. I was in real pain—but by that time I was no longer suffering. The accomplishment of having run 26-plus miles thrilled me. I had a sense of vitality and a significant increase in self-esteem. I was buoyed in my success at having accomplished my established goal.

REAL PAIN

All pain is real pain—even if it seems imagined or exaggerated to the rest of us. Almost all my patients come to see me because of real pain.

Ninety percent of these patients respond by getting better. They go back to sports, play, and work. They do not experience long-term (chronic) pain, nor do they seem to suffer.

**Pain is perfect misery . . .
"the worst of evils."**
—John Milton, *Paradise Lost*

Sufferers, however, are very different. I can spot them immediately. They typically have "total body anguish," appearing depressed, discouraged, and distrustful. They generally don't like their work or life situation. Sufferers are usually passive about their contribution to their suffering and may become angry if others or "the system" does not do something for them. As patients, they usually come to the doctor with someone else who validates their pain, for example, a suffering adult comes with his or her mother, or an injured worker comes with his or her spouse. They will be taking several medications.

These patients can try my soul, though I sometimes recognize myself in them. Scott Peck in *In Search of Stones* states, "You can never get enough of what you don't really need." No matter how much attention I lavish on some of them, it never seems to be enough. I want desperately to help them and know that they are truly suffering.

Because sufferers are so difficult to treat, it is truly a joy when I am able to help them recover. Occasionally I have to either push or drag them along the road to health. The process is never easy. It takes longer and is more expensive and exhausting than any of us would like. But knowing that every person is a God-created being of infinite worth, deserving dignity and respect, is motivation to keep going.

OTHER KINDS OF SUFFERING

Physical pain is an issue to which each of us is sensitive and responsive. It seems to pale, however, when compared to the anguish offered by some of life's less-welcome events:

◆ Separation from those near and dear to us
◆ Death of someone we love
◆ Mental and emotional pain
◆ Financial disaster leading to bankruptcy, homelessness, hunger, or ill health due to deprivation
◆ Spiritual death and hopelessness

Approximately 29 years ago we adopted Heather when she was only three days old. An amazing series of events led to her adoption.

On a Tuesday morning I called an attorney friend of ours who happened to also be legal counsel to an adoption agency. Heather had been born that morning. By Friday of the same week, we were walking out of a hospital with her in our arms. Our lives have been tightly intertwined ever since. She is better and more wonderful than we could have ever dreamed. She is brilliant, beautiful, talented, intuitive, sensitive, and kind.

Heather has always been happy to be our daughter; we usually forget she's adopted. At age 22, with our encouragement and support, she began a search for her birth mother. It was an exciting time. Aarlie and I could hardly wait to meet the person who had contributed so much to our incredible daughter. We were anxious for her to see how well things had worked out for the baby she had relinquished so many years before.

The search agency was efficient, and the birth mother was located within a few weeks. Heather wrote a letter to her. It was an incredible effort, telling about her life, faith, dreams, and abilities, and her desire to meet and know her birth mother.

As she waited for a response, all the natural questions were going through her mind and heart. Who are you? Who is my birth father? But the biggest questions were, Will you accept or reject me—will you welcome me or send me away? Why didn't you keep me? Will we like each other? Will you be proud of me, and I of you?

Weeks and weeks went by. Finally, a thick letter came in the mail bearing the search agency's return address. Heather knew it was from her birth mother. She called and told us her plan. She was going to take a shower, fix her hair, put on her prettiest dress, and go alone to her favorite spot in a nearby park. There she would open the letter and "meet" her birth mother.

The letter was full of information. The mother gave a brief history of herself, a detailed narrative of her relationship with Heather's birth father, and why she felt she had to give her up for adoption. She told her everything she knew about the birth father. She wrote of her recent Christian conversion and expressed happiness that Heather was a Christian and that her life was going so well. She enclosed a recent picture of herself and revealed that Heather had two half brothers.

But the things Heather needed and wanted most were denied. Her birth mother could not and would not meet her, even at a neutral clandestine location at no expense to her. The reason was that her husband and family did not know about Heather's birth, and she was afraid to tell them.

Heather experienced deep rejection. She cried. We cried. Even as I write this many years later, I'm crying again.

This kind of suffering is not like sore legs and muscles; it affects the total being—mind, soul, and body. Every nerve ending seems raw. Every thought is painful. Every cell in the body aches, and every function of the soul is labored. Divorce, death, a runaway child, separation from those we love, all rejection and loss must feel somewhat like this.

**Nothing that happens in our lives is
wasted energy. God in some way will find
a way to put it to good
use sometime, somewhere.**
—Joseph F. Girzone

In Heather's life as the weeks, months, and years have passed, the pain and suffering have diminished but remain lodged never too far below the surface—deep enough so life does not stand still, deep enough that she is able to remain effective and active, but readily available as a graphic template of loss and rejection to be applied to other risky ventures.

It is my observation that Heather's losses and separations in relationships with others have been made more difficult and more severe in part, at least, by the loss and suffering she experienced in the rejection by her birth mother.

**Suffering and pain are part
of the human experience
—no exceptions and no exemptions.**

GARY / JIM / JOHN / WAYNE

Gary, Jim, John, and Wayne were all close friends of mine who died too young. Each played important roles in my life, and since their deaths virtually overlapped, I was in a constant crush of grief and separation for several consecutive years.

Three of the four left two young children in the wake of their passage. They all left widows. None had reached their potential: life was wrenched, twisted, and extracted out of them despite radiation; chemotherapy; bone marrow transplants; prayer; healing services; family-church-friend support; positive, optimistic attitudes; counseling; and hope.

They had every reason to live and no apparent reason to die except that each had incurable cancer.

- ◆ Jim fought to the last moment in the midst of one more treatment and one more attempt at a bone marrow transplant.
- ◆ John seemed to have no options or treatment left, and he quietly and bravely crossed from death to life.
- ◆ Gary opted to "go fishing" after his third relapse. In many ways, that decision was the most courageous of them all.
- ◆ Wayne, as the oldest, set the example of dignity in death.

At their funerals, I spoke at the request of their families. We rejoiced in the hope of new life and the liberation of each of them from pain and suffering. But the words at times felt hollow in the face of great sorrow.

**A diamond is a piece of coal
that has suffered.**
—Joseph F. Girzone

SCHIZOPHRENIC

My brother-in-law Glenn was well liked, smart, handsome, and president of the student body. He was the third of five wonderful children. In the eighth grade he was diagnosed with paranoid schizophrenia. The disease caused a marked loss of functional living skills. Tormented by voices and delusions, he has been in and out of private and state hospitals and is now in an assisted living environment. Unable to hold a job, he never really had a chance to dream a future or to plan his own path in life. Glenn's father died having not seen his son healthy for nearly 40 years.

The stories regarding Glenn are beyond cataloging: funny, bizarre, sad, and scary. In them there is much pain.

WHERE IS GOD?

Why didn't God demonstrate miraculous power in Heather's request? Why didn't He heal Gary, Jim, John, or Wayne? Why has He allowed Glenn to continue suffering? Is God really a God of goodness and of power?

C. S. Lewis writes in *The Problem of Pain*, "We want, in fact, not so much a father in heaven as a grandfather in heaven—a senile benevolence who, as they say, 'likes to see young people enjoying themselves,' and whose plan for the universe was simply that it might be truly said at the end of each day, 'A good time was had by all.'" Lewis goes on to say, "If God were good, He would wish to make His creatures perfectly happy, and if God were almighty, He would be able to do what He wished. But the creatures are not happy. Therefore, God lacks either goodness, or power, or both. This is the problem of pain, in its simplest form."

And yet Christians choose to believe that God is *both* good and all-powerful. A. W. Tozer writes in *The Knowledge of the Holy*:

> That God is good is taught or implied on every page of the Bible and must be received as an article of faith as impregnable as the throne of God. It is a foundation stone for all sound thought about God and is necessary to moral sanity. To allow that God could be other than good is to deny the validity of all thought and end in the negation of every moral judgment. If God is not good, then there can be no distinction between kindness and cruelty, and heaven can be hell, and hell heaven.
>
> The goodness of God is the drive behind all the blessings He daily bestows upon us. God created us because He felt good in His heart and He redeemed us for the same reason.

Tozer goes on to say that sin, time, and rebellion have made us timid and self-conscious in our approach to believing that God is good. These years of rebellion against God have bred in us a fear that is not easily overcome. Tozer says we ask the questions, "If I come to God, how will He act toward me? What kind of disposition has He? What will I find Him to be like?"

The answer is that He will be found to be exactly like Jesus. "He that has seen me," says Jesus, "has seen the Father." From Jesus we learn how God acts toward people.

My family still prays for a miracle for Glenn, but not with great intensity. We have grown weary—our eyes are dry; our hearts fear to hope. But even though our bringing him to God has not resulted in the cure we had hoped for, Glenn experiences physical health and some moments of peace and clarity.

Certainly we have become very aware of the hand of God working through Glenn to touch and teach us. When we drive through the inner city and see homeless people, the unemployed, or the disadvantaged, we recognize people just like Glenn. When we see people, churches, institutions, and government agencies giving time, money, and programs, we think of Glenn. And when we think of heaven and wholeness and recognize his obvious desire to be a godly person, we see a healthy Glenn with a sound mind and freedom from tormenting voices and thoughts. This world is not all there is. Heaven is our hope. Scripture tells us that the sufferings of this present time cannot in any way be compared with the glory and the beauty and the wonder that we shall experience in heaven (see Rom. 8:18).

"[Any discussion] on suffering which says nothing of heaven is leaving out almost the whole of one side of the account," C. S. Lewis reminds us in *The Problem of Pain*. "Scripture and tradition habitually put the joys of heaven into the scale against the sufferings of earth, and no solution of the problem of pain which does not do so can be called a Christian one. . . . But either there is pie in the sky or there is not. If there is not, then Christianity is false, for this doctrine is woven into the whole fabric. If there is, then this truth, like any other, must be faced, whether it is useful at political meetings or not."

So it is to "the pie in the sky" that we turn. The Bible, Christian tradition, church belief, and our own understanding of God validates that we are not abstract creatures in God's eyes but that we are individuals created and loved by God and redeemed to spend eternity with Him in heaven. In fact, a special mansion and place are being made for each of us. Glenn's may be one of the nicest of all, for he certainly has suffered much in this life. I hope he has open house from time to time.

THE BLAME GAME

Many of us have asked *why* at times. I certainly have, though seldom with any real bitterness. For the most part, Christians seem to understand that pain is part of life. Is there an explanation for our seeming complacency? It's certainly not that God cannot take a little blame now and again: He's big enough to handle it. Is it that we recognize our own complicity with suffering? Or our impatience? Our dissatisfaction with differential results? Timothy exhorts us that "everyone who wants to live a godly life in Christ Jesus will be persecuted" (2 Tim. 3:12). Perhaps we are beginning to accept that there is some value in suffering.

Paul Brand states in his and Phillip Yancey's book *Pain, the Gift Nobody Wants*, "Thank God for inventing pain! I don't think he could have done a better job. It is beautiful!"

"Pain is not an afterthought, or God's great goof," he continues. "Rather, it reveals a marvelous design that serves our bodies well. Pain is as essential to a normal life, it could be argued, as eyesight or even good circulation. Without pain . . . our lives would be fraught with danger, and devoid of many basic pleasures."

Regardless of its value to us, pain certainly insists upon being attended to. "God whispers to us in our pleasures, speaks in our conscience, but shouts in our pains," Lewis writes in *The Problem of Pain*. "It is His megaphone to rouse a deaf world."

Scripture confirms it: "Consider it pure joy, my brothers, whenever you face trials of many kinds, because you know that the testing of your faith develops perseverance. Perseverance must finish its work so that you may be mature and complete, not lacking anything" (James 1:2-4).

Human beings are not omniscient or omnipotent. All accumulated knowledge doesn't even register on the scale when compared to the infinite knowledge of God. How is it that we presume to tell God what to do or to blame Him if He doesn't follow our instructions?

Frank Minirth and Paul Meier in their book *Happiness Is a Choice* write:

> Why God didn't make any of us humans perfect we don't know, but we trust the God of all wisdom, love, and justice to make the correct ultimate decisions. To be angry at God for not being more "humane" is naive, arrogant, and pompous. In our practice we run into many immature individuals who naively think they are wiser and kinder than God. They think God makes mistakes. But man looks at the pain of a moment, while God looks at the joys of an eternity. Man is capable of empathizing with the pain

of depression. God not only empathizes with man's pain (Christ suffered the painful death of the cross), but rejoices in the growth toward maturity that is occurring in the individual who is responsibly working his way out of a depression.

Once we did have a perfect world without pain, suffering, and loss. But man and woman in a world without suffering chose to go against God. We have done the same thing time and time again. Let us learn instead to choose those blessings offered by God rather than the cruel fruits of our own indulgence.

FORWARD-LOOKING RESPONSE

The ability to convert suffering into a healthy and positive response is a grand and giant step toward wholeness.

In *Pain, the Gift Nobody Wants,* Brand and Yancey write:

Circumstances, whether fortunate or unfortunate, are morally neutral. They simply are what they are: what matters is how we respond to them. Good and evil, in the moral sense, do not reside in things, but always in persons. What we are confronted with, as caregivers, lovers, brothers, friends, neighbors and pastors, mothers and teachers, is the obligation to help people channel suffering and use it as a transforming agent.

Suffering is not beneficial in itself, and we must always fight against it. However, in an imperfect world, suffering can

- ◆ remind us we need to make positive responses to bad situations;
- ◆ help us learn not to blame ourselves for the full extent of our pain;
- ◆ give us a more acute sense of joy, good, and right;
- ◆ help us to know that pain and suffering cannot control our minds, spirits, and inner selves;
- ◆ pull our focus off the material and physical, and toward the spiritual, social, emotional, and mental;
- ◆ turn us to God. We do not need to be fatalistic but know that with God's help there can be a better tomorrow. A God who can create our universe and us can calm the troubled seas of our lives and can give us a new start.

COPING WITH PAIN, SUFFERING, AND LOSS

Psychological Intervention

Pain, loss, suffering, and psychological distress are often inseparable. Dealing with chronic pain leads to depression, anger, anxiety, bitterness, sleeplessness, helplessness, instability, decreased energy, financial worries, lifestyle changes, treatment schedules, loss of family structure, and so on. These things in turn lead to more loss and more suffering.

All of us have experienced frustration when we can't find our car keys, lose our appointment book, or experience minor crises. Imagine the feelings you would experience if your entire life was turned upside down, and you can begin to see why specific intervention is sometimes necessary.

There are many ways to get help:

1. *Individual therapy.* A friend, pastor, social worker, psychologist, or psychiatrist could be a good therapist. In individual therapy we can begin to identify maladaptive and negative thoughts. We can also begin to dispute irrational thinking, learn distracting techniques, and work on developing increased social support skills.

2. *Group therapy.* There are grief groups, loss groups, chronic pain groups—groups that would probably fit most needs or aspects of suffering, pain, and loss. Group therapy can assist us to develop restructuring, adaptive coping skills and to direct our behaviors in a more positive manner.

3. *Treatment of depression/anxiety.* Medications, professional help, and physical activity are viable options.

4. *Cognitive behavioral therapy.* This helps us see problems as manageable instead of overwhelming. We learn to reframe a problem into small components in which we have control. This can help us become actively involved in treatment choices and solutions.

5. *Pain clinics.* If your pain has a physical component and you have been through the usual processes and programs and have come up to an end point in dealing with it, then you may benefit from a pain clinic at a large center with a multidisciplinary approach to pain.

Physical Intervention

Pain and physical dependence on medication can result in muscular weakness, deconditioning, and stiffness. All these factors lead to the need for

1. *Physical activity.* Get a personal trainer, join a fitness club, and find a friend to be accountable to/with.

2. *Relaxation training.* Residual muscle spasms and tensions are exceedingly high in conditions of pain, suffering, and loss. We need to develop new reflexes and responses to create relief. Biofeedback, electromyography, thermal biofeedback techniques, music therapy, and other techniques can be useful in providing a new and positive environment for relief.

Spiritual Intervention

1. *Positive faith.* A belief system in the God of the universe is vital to the spiritual intervention we all need when coping with pain and loss. Seek the presence of the Holy. Allow the still, small voice of God to speak to your innermost being.

2. *Prayer.* Dependence on the Divine in all societies through all the ages has been significant in ensuring recovery and coping.

3. *Bible study.* An incredible number of Bible verses of promise, hope, help, and health are available to help us with our suffering and loss.

4. *Religious activities.* Church attendance, small groups, and Bible study fellowships are important spiritual tools for recovery. Be involved in worship services. Sing songs of faith.

5. *Hope of heaven.* This life is not all there is. We are only pilgrims passing through. Our eternal home will be just that—eternal.

"The resurrection [of Jesus] and its victory over death brought a decisive new word to the vocabulary of pain and suffering: temporary," writes Paul Brand and Phillip Yancey in *Pain, the Gift Nobody Wants.* "Jesus Christ holds out the startling promise of an afterlife without pain. Whatever anguish we feel now will not last. The Christian's final hope, then, is hope in a painless future, with God."

While most of us have not experienced a great deal of pain, loss, or suffering, we all know those who have. It is important to recognize that our joys have been numerous. For these we say thanks, and for all those days and events yet ahead, we say yes, realizing we will need and receive grace and strength.

DOCTOR'S ORDERS: RX FOR PAIN AND SUFFERING

▶ Remember: pain, suffering, and loss are morally neutral. Their presence is not as important as your response to them.

▶ We all face pain, suffering, and loss—these, too, will pass.

▶ Deal with your pain at a physical, emotional, and spiritual level. The struggle will make you stronger.

If we do not change our direction, we are likely to end up where we are going.

—Chinese proverb

CHAPTER 4

A WORD FROM THE PROFESSOR . . .

HOPE

I remember a verse quoted often around our farmhouse when I was a child:

> *Hitch your wagon to a star.*
> *Keep your seat, and there you are.*

In this context my sister, brother, and I contemplated our futures. For a while I wanted to become a cattle auctioneer. Nothing matched the excitement of accompanying my dad to the Ontario (Oregon) Cattle Auction. Later I aspired to become a journalist. Our town's weekly newspaper, the *Ontario Argus Observer*, caught my attention with its reporting of people, places, and events.

I never felt destined to stay on our small dairy farm. The future seemed filled with exciting options. It never occurred to me that I would not attend college. My mother would not permit even a passing mention of skipping college in order to pursue some other career path. Perhaps she still felt the pain of the deprivation that necessitated her withdrawal from West Texas State after only nine weeks. She would do better by her children.

Another bit of wisdom taught on that small 65-acre farm comes to mind, "It's better to aim for a star and miss than to aim for the barn door and hit." As our parents embedded dreams for the future in us, they served notice that no sacrifice would be too great for them to enable those dreams to come true. Among other things, Mother took employment at Ontario's Eastside Laundry doing washing and ironing. I was impressed then but have become increasingly more appreciative with the passing years of the sacrifice my parents made to guarantee their children a college education.

YOU GOTTA HAVE HOPE

"There's enough suffering to go around"—this is a phrase that captures volumes about the human experience. One of my graduate school professors, W. T. Purkiser, commented in his book *When You Get to the End of Yourself*, "Life can be terribly hard for most people some of the time and for some people most of the time. There is no easy way to explain this. We cannot understand why the dark night of the soul should come."

Over time, difficulties, defeats, disappointments, and other like realities accumulate within our lives. We can become so full of darkness that there seems to be no room in us for hope. Hopelessness is the admission that whatever I do does not matter and will not change my circumstances.

In *Legacy of the Heart: The Spiritual Advantages of a Painful Childhood*, Wayne Muller tells about visiting an elderly Hispanic carpenter who was dying of AIDS (Acquired Immune Deficiency Syndrome). Muller had been informed that the man needed to process his "issues" about dying. Muller wrote:

> When I arrived, he didn't want to talk about his "issues" at all. "You're a minister, aren't you?" he asked me. I replied that I was. "Why don't you just pray with me?" So I sat and prayed with him. . . .
>
> When we finished praying, I finally questioned him about his illness. Why, I asked, did he think he had AIDS, why did he feel he was given this illness? He thought about my question, turned slowly to me, and said, "So I could have more time to think about Jesus."
>
> Who knew why he had AIDS, whose fault it was, or who had given it to him? All he could do, in the depth of weariness and fear, was listen for the merciful voice of God. He was dying in great pain. But in that excruciating moment he was listening for a deeper

healing, for the love and faith that would fill his heart with grace as he made his way home.

The God of all grace is the Source of our hope regardless of how the odds are stacked against us. But when I cave in and believe that nothing I do will influence the outcome of my situation, I become hopeless; I am a victim of my circumstances, and I develop a mind-set that leads to depression and despair.

My neighbor is a husband and a father of four young children who will find himself unemployed at the end of this month. Recently he told me that he will sell his home and move closer to extended family. Such a decision is not unusual in these times of economic uncertainty. Although he does not consider the move an ideal scenario for his family, many favorable outcomes may result. As we visited, though, I was struck with my friend's despair. "I guess it's just as easy to tread water over there as it is here," he commented glumly. He assumed that his actions would have little or no effect on the desired outcome.

When we hope, we wish for something with the expectation that it might happen. When we are hopeless, we regard our situation as one that defies solution. Psychologist Martin Seligman in *Learned Optimism* calls the feeling "helplessness." He notes, "Helplessness is a state of affairs in which nothing you choose to do affects what happens to you."

Too many of us are locked into believing that what we do will not influence what happens in our future. For some, this attitude is precipitated by circumstances of our own making. But often, unsuspecting persons find themselves victims of crimes, accidents, natural disasters, or disease. Each day the evening news reporters recite the names of places and persons jerked into the battle where despair challenges hope.

On July 17, 1996, TWA Flight 800 went down following takeoff from New York City's John F. Kennedy International Airport. In the aftermath, how meaningful is the concept of hope to the family members of the 230 people who were on board? More specifically, what about the residents of the small community of Mountoursville, Pennsylvania, who had 21 persons from the high school French club on the flight? What will become the "collective community psyche" of Mountoursville as they process the bereavement and the "starting over" required to survive such a tragedy? Is the word *hope* a hollow concept for them or an anchor for rebuilding their community?

Hopelessness and wholeness are incompatible traveling com-
panions. Hope about one's circumstances, future, options, and the
ability to choose one's attitudes regardless of the degree of adversity is
a necessary dimension of wholeness. It is true that there are many
things outside of my control—my eye color, the future price of agricul-
tural commodities, and a hurricane sweeping along the coastline of
the Carolinas. But there are many circumstances within my control—
one of those being my ability to choose my attitudes and reactions to
all circumstances.

Hope believes in possibilities. Hope declares that there is the potential of a future. Hope leans into the inevitability of change, knowing that there are always choices. Hope enables us to avoid the de-
struction of unchecked despair, depression, and helplessness.

A BIG FOUR-LETTER WORD

Inside each of us is a perspective on life. We understand hope as one
of those gut feelings that sometimes defies logical explanation. A
hopeful person deals with the following questions differently than
does a hopeless person:

Will my efforts make any difference?
Will I be able to survive these challenges?
Will this crisis ever pass?
Am I and my family going to be OK?
Will I be able to cope?
Can I influence the shape of my future?
Do I have options from which I may choose?

Seligman notes that the way we think about life enlarges or di-
minishes the amount of control we experience. Our thoughts, he suggests, are not merely reactions to events but change agents influencing
what occurs. He writes:

> For example, if we think we are helpless to make a differ-
> ence in what our children become, we will be paralyzed when
> dealing with this facet of our lives. The very thought "Nothing I
> do matters" prevents us from acting. . . .
> Twenty-five years of study has convinced me that if we ha-
> bitually believe, as does the pessimist, that misfortune is our

fault, is enduring, and will undermine everything we do, more of it will befall us than if we believe otherwise. I am convinced that if we are in the grip of this view, we will get depressed easily, we will accomplish less than our potential, and we will even get physically sick more often. Pessimistic prophecies are self-fulfilling.

ASSESSING AND SHAPING MY STORY

Our culture is obsessed with the theme of "self." The achievement of self-esteem, self-actualization, self-acceptance, or self-development has become both a right and a national preoccupation. Americans claim a right to sufficient food, adequate shelter, protection from the elements, free education, and basic health care. In addition, there is this new "right"—that of the care and development of one's "self."

Consider the way we view our work. Years ago there was an emphasis on the extrinsic nature of labor, that is, we worked in order to earn income to support our families. Now we demand more. As a culture occupied with self, we believe our jobs must have larger meaning. We ask, "Is my work a statement about me and what I value?" or "Do I find my work fulfilling?" If my answers are negative, I am expected to quit my job. No one should work only for extrinsic reasons.

A DIFFERENT PERSPECTIVE: GOOD OUT OF BAD

Wayne Muller's provocative book *Legacy of the Heart: The Spiritual Advantages of a Painful Childhood* is a book for our time, reflecting our zealous commitment to self-reflection and self-esteem. In it, Muller points to the multitude of self-support groups in our culture as an indicator of what we regard important. He observes that these groups help us explore the social environments in which we were reared and their presumed deficiencies. Some of the more popular groups assist adults reared in homes in which there was alcoholism or drug abuse. Other groups organize around adult survivors of domestic violence.

Muller helps us take a different look at the deprived and dysfunctional homes in which people have been reared. He understands the loss many experienced as children but raises the prospect of the "advantages" of a bad childhood.

Muller does not deny that some grow up in terrible conditions. But he believes that a person is not a condition or a victim or a diagnosis or a label, even if self-assigned. He says that too often one's life narrative is built on the limitations of the past:

> After many years, our habitual ways of seeing ourselves become so chronic that we can hardly imagine any others. We are no longer simply a child, a human being; we have become the Unloved, the Vulnerable, the Disappointed One, the Abandoned, the Misunderstood, the Deprived, the Terribly Broken. Waking up in the morning and getting ready for the day, *we put on our story* [emphasis added] like an old bathrobe and a soft pair of slippers. We are so accustomed to introducing ourselves as the victim of our story, we actually feel ambivalent about whether or not we can really change—or even want to. Our very life becomes a familiar, droning habit.

We each have strengths, regardless of the scars from difficult childhoods and other traumatizing experiences. These scars may go deep into our emotions, memories, and psyche. But we can rewrite our stories, contends Muller:

> Take your time. . . . The scars of childhood have long shadows deep in the heart, and are not readily let go of. All healing requires gentleness, attention, and care. But keep in mind that you need not repair, reconstruct, or remake yourself into someone else. Your practice is simply to rewaken what is already wise and strong, to claim what is deep and true within you, to rediscover your own intuition, to find your inner balance, and to reaffirm your intrinsic wholeness in the eyes of God.

GRACE: THE SOURCE OF HOPE

Bubbling below the surface in our discussion on hope is the theological concept of grace. Grace declares that innate within all persons is the presence of the Divine.

The presence of divinity within us is the operative power of God giving us insight for attitudes and actions. This inner influence of God enables us to walk in ways pleasing to Him. We are made in His image and endowed with His presence. The quest to own and develop our

spirituality is part of what it means to be human and an important element in wholeness.

Grace is the loving and shaping influence of God operative within
our lives. Grace is the active re-creating influence of God drawing us to
come into alignment with sovereignty's intentions and the potentialities
with which we have been endowed. Theologian Mildred Bangs
Wynkoop in *Foundations of Wesleyan-Arminian Theology* linked quotations
from Wiley and Bernard to capture the significance of this theme. She
wrote:

> We may say then, that man was endowed with certain pow-
> ers known as the natural image . . . [which is] uneffaced and inef-
> faceable, and exists in every human being. This natural likeness to
> God is inalienable. . . . This first element of the divine image man
> can never lose until he ceases to be a man. St. Bernard well said
> that it could not be burned out, even in hell.

BIDDEN OR NOT, GOD IS PRESENT

Barbara and I purchased a beautiful ceramic plaque for the front entry
wall of our house. On it is the message that hung over the front door
of Carl Jung's house in Zurich, Switzerland: "Bidden or not, God is
present." Later this message, written in Latin, was placed on Jung's
tombstone. Jung (1875-1961) noted that this declaration of faith about
the presence of God pointed to Ps. 111:10: "The fear of the LORD is the
beginning of wisdom." Jung would concur with those who declare the
reality of grace, that wherever we go, with whomever we speak, and
whatever the situation, God is already present.

To be made in the image of God and to have a spark of divinity
within gives us cause for optimism—the optimism of grace. Each of us
is designed to cope, to find meaning, to survive and thrive as a moral
being. We were created to become, to recognize our purpose, and to
enter into some cause worthy of our efforts. We were designed so that
deep within there is a sense of connectedness with the wise and gracious Creator of the universe.

MEANINGLESS GOD TALK OR REALITY?

Is this "grace stuff" simply meaningless God talk—gobbledygook?
Does it match the reality of human experience? Recently I attended a

meeting sponsored by the Idaho Department of Health and Welfare. It was a "community conve sation" about projected changes in welfare benefits. During the evening we divided into small discussion groups. One member in my group, a woman in her early 40s, reported that all three of her teenage children are handicapped, one with multiple handicaps. She noted that each school day is a disaster waiting to happen. She cannot find anyone willing to provide child care for her youngsters so she can work outside the home. The two-year limits and decreased monthly cash benefits we were discussing are more than political posturing for her. Given her circumstances, welfare benefits equal survival. How do we measure the meaning of grace in the life of this woman and her family?

I hope she was listening to NBC News's coverage of the Olympics in Atlanta July 24, 1996. If so, she heard a message of grace. The closing feature of the Olympics coverage was a blitz of scenes of key events of the day displaying both victory and defeat. The musical background was a choir singing several verses of John Newton's famous hymn "Amazing Grace." One verse declares,

> *The Lord has promised good to me;*
> *His word my hope secures.*
> *He will my shield and portion be*
> *As long as life endures.*

God places deep within each of us an invitation to hope. Mysterious ways in which God works the simple hearing of these words bring reflection, comfort, and momentary invitation to hope.

WE MAY CHOOSE GRACE

As wonderful and important as divine grace is, we must place proper emphasis upon human participation, choice, and accountability. John Wesley captured this balance in his statement: "Sufficient grace in all, irresistible grace in none."

Let's pull the strands together and declare the privilege of hope through grace. We have been made in the image of God. Active within us, as grace, is the influence of God giving us the privilege of making decisions for right and good. The merciful God of the universe will not give up on us. Throughout history God has shown that He is un-

willing to junk the human project. Professor Michael Lodahl writes in
The Story of God about God's commitment to His creation:

> God persists, and this persistence we call grace, for grace
> refers, in part, to His unwillingness ever to give up on us. Perhaps
> God has thrown himself so enthusiastically into the task of creating
> that to quit on it would be to deny His own character as Creator.

Lodahl develops the idea further. He suggests that we sometimes envision history as God playing a giant game of solitaire. In this
context God lays out all the options and then chooses a sequence of
events. However, if we accept the idea that a God of grace is involved,
we dare to believe that the forming of history is dynamic and interac-
tive with humans as meaningful, although sometimes badly mistaken,
actors. So, it is not a divine Being engaged in a game of solitaire but a
divine Being involved with us in the unchartered course of unfolding
history. We take confidence that the God of grace will "hang in there"
with us regardless.

God persists in our behalf and in behalf of the course of history
common to all of us The sovereign One is best understood as "the
God of fresh starts and new beginnings." This translates into *hope* for
vulnerable and mortal humans. The words of Jeremiah, spoken to his
fellow citizens in exile, is a universal message of hope for each person,
regardless of era or nation of citizenship:

> Thus says the LORD: After seventy years are completed at
> Babylon, I will visit you and perform My good word toward you,
> and cause you to return to this place. For I know the thoughts that I
> think toward you, says the LORD, thoughts of peace and not of evil,
> to give you a future and a hope *(Jer. 29:10-11, NKJV)*.

The chapter you're reading begins with a Chinese proverb: "If
we do not change our direction, we are likely to end up where we are
going." Human beings always have choices. God has graced each of
us so we may make decisions about life's perspectives. We can change
our direction and choose hope.

Choice is the avenue to wholeness. We can choose to make
habits—or to break habits. We can choose to increase the importance
we place on some activities. Likewise, we can choose to decrease the

priority given to other activities. My children, Karen and Tim, will document that my favorite "parental lecture" during their childhood and adolescent years was "Attitude Is a Choice." Hope, I have come to believe, is also a choice available to us because of the grace of God.

THE PROF'S HOMEWORK ASSIGNMENT: NEWNESS

I heard a quotation of Christian believers attributed to Augustine: "We're Easter men and Easter women, and Hallelujah is our song." The story of Jesus' resurrection from the dead is the consummate illustration that we serve a God of fresh starts and new beginnings.

Locate a favorite study Bible and look for the theme of newness. The gospel of Christ is full of newness—fresh starts and new beginnings. Expand on the following list of the newness theme found in the New Testament.

▶ A new message

▶ A new heart

▶ A new heaven and a new earth

▶ A new (second) birth

▶ A new fellowship (family) of believers

▶ A new spiritual (glorified) body
(Add other ideas.)

Take hope. God wants to do fresh new things within us, among us, and through us.

Prayer is friendship with God. . . . Prayer is listening as well as speaking, receiving as well as asking; and its deepest mood is friendship held in reverence.

—George Buttrick

CHAPTER 5

A WORD FROM THE DOCTOR . . .
PRAYER

s a child, I cannot remember one significant circumstance in which my family did not pray. We prayed for every conceivable person and situation. We prayed for good attitudes and unselfish lifestyles. We prayed for plentiful crops and healthy cows. We prayed about everything.

I believe those prayers have made a great difference in the outcome of many situations. But probably the biggest effect they had on my life was impressing on me the fact that the sovereign God is accessible. He knows my name, where I live, what I think, and how I feel. He listens to my heart, knowing my *real* prayer even when I don't. He answers every prayer in conformity with His will.

> Is any one of you in trouble? He should pray. Is anyone happy? Let him sing songs of praise. Is any one of you sick? He should call the elders of the church to pray over him and anoint him with oil in the name of the Lord. And the prayer offered in faith will make the sick person well; the Lord will raise him up. If he has sinned, he will be forgiven. Therefore confess your sins to each other and pray for each other so that you may be healed. The prayer of a righteous man is powerful and effective *(James 5:13-16).*

When I was an orthopedic resident at the University of Washington in Seattle, I was given a one-year assignment to a children's hospital in Spokane, Washington. Patients would come to the hospital and stay for weeks, sometimes months, while they were treated. There was no formal religious program or Sunday church service for the patients. So with the help of my wife, friends, and our church's young people, we started a Sunday service. It was wonderful. The nursing staff loved it. The patients enjoyed the variety it brought to their week.

I will never forget one particular patient named Patty. Patty was a 13-year-old female with a double-curve deformity from scoliosis. She had undergone a back fusion 12 months earlier, but it had become obvious that the fusion was not successful. She still had low back pain with motion of the lumbar spine. Surgery would be necessary to graft the bone together.

The Sunday before Patty's surgery, we prayed for her, asking that God's miracle of healing would occur in her life. We assumed that healing would be accomplished by surgery.

But the next week when we took Patty to surgery, we found that the miracle had already occurred. When we operated on her back, we found a solid spine. She did not need a fusion and bone grafting. As a young surgeon enamored with what surgery could do for people, I was reminded that all healing is a miracle.

As a practitioner of medicine and surgery, I am not only a healer but a *pray-er*. Without the healing power of God, my surgical repairs and incisions wouldn't heal, the bones I set wouldn't knit back together, and my "healing arts" wouldn't exist.

A HEALER AND A PRAY-ER

This principle of pray-er and healer was brought home very dramatically to me recently. My patient this time was a healthy, adolescent female athlete. She was referred to me by coaches and by former patients I had treated successfully. She wanted to see a "knee/sports medicine doctor" who could fix her knee and get her ready for basketball in just six months.

It seemed routine, easy, predictable—I had repaired isolated anterior cruciate ligament tears hundreds of times. But when I took this young athlete to surgery, every step of the procedure was difficult. Vi-

sualization by the arthroscope was poor, portal placement was not
ideal, the equipment seemed to have constant technical problems, har-
vesting the graft was tough, and placement of the new ligament was
even worse. The fixation of the new ligament was marginal, my highly
skilled assistants seemed inept, the operating room got hotter and hotter, and on and on it went.

I finally ended the surgery having done all I could do. I was discouraged and disappointed. I wasn't optimistic about the outcome. I
prayed, "God, You and I are partners in life and in this practice. Please
step forward and take over. I need Your help. Please heal this patient's
knee and give her a good result." Each time she came to my mind
(which was often), I would pray for a great result. God answered my
prayer, and the girl's knee was fine.

Would Patty at Spokane Children's Hospital have been healed
without prayers? Was the good result of the surgery on the knee of the
athlete a result of my desperate plea for help? Some would say we'll
never know. But for me, both cases were dramatic demonstrations of
the power and providence of the supernatural.

"The history of mankind will probably show that no people has
ever risen above its religion, and no religion has ever been greater
than (its) idea of God," wrote A. W. Tozer in *The Knowledge of the Holy*.
A magnificent and lofty concept of God is essential if we are to experience real power in prayer. Even so, prayer is an everyday activity for
ordinary folks. It is not magic or an exclusive ritual reserved for specialists in religion.

A person's body, mind, and soul blend into a unified integrated
whole by the development of our spiritual being. The equation for
wholeness might look as follows: $Sp^n (P+I+E+So)$ = wholeness. Sp =
spiritual elements; P = physical strength; I = intellectual vigor; E =
emotional stability; So = social competence; n = 2 or more. The product is wholeness.

In the equation, the spiritual element is the most powerful as it is
both a multiplication and exponential factor. A small increase in the
spiritual element (such as prayer, religious activity, belief, faith, reading the Holy Scriptures) results in big dividends. Even though physical strength, intellectual vigor, emotional stability, and social competence are important, they don't carry the same significance.

Have you noticed that when we discipline ourselves to control one aspect of our lives, discipline tends to spill over into other areas and we ap important benefits? For example, becoming physically fit by regular workouts and a good diet may allow us to apply the same self-discipline to begin a regular prayer-meditation time. We cannot compartmentalize our personhood into separate entities.

GOD IS GOOD FOR YOU

Fifteen years ago I began experiencing numbness on the left side of my body and significant weakness on the right side. I immediately consulted a neurologist, who, after evaluating me, told me I had a cervical spine tumor, or multiple sclerosis. He scheduled me for a myelogram and a computerized axial tomography (CAT) scan to differentiate the diagnosis. The tests were to be done the next day.

That evening before the tests, I began counting my blessings: Aarlie was 39 years old; I was 43. Our five children ranged in age from 3 to 16. But the blessings seemed to fade as the words "tumor or multiple sclerosis" echoed in my mind. How could I do surgery? How would I help raise my kids and send them to college? What if I died? Who would read stories to my kids, teach them to ski, show them how to change a tire? Who would wrestle with them at night? I knew Aarlie would be OK. We had had over 18 years of a great marriage, more than many people get in an entire lifetime.

I prayed that night. The sky was clear, the heavens were open, and stars dotted the blackness. Hot tears streamed down my face as I begged for *my* God to come to *my* world. I prayed that I would be well and live long enough to help raise my children and know the joy of seeing them grow up.

Suddenly my mind was calmed, and I began to feel hope. The healing process had begun. I went back into the house with a sense of confidence that everything was going to be all right.

Tests the next day did not reveal anything definitive. But the next 5 to 10 years proved to be a time of slow healing. At first I could not walk without a foot drop on the right. I started jogging because I knew that a fit body was best for me and would make me more productive and healthier. The first day, I ran 1 mile out and 1 mile back. It took me 20 minutes, and I had to high-step on the right side to get my foot through without dragging my toe, but it was a celebration of life and healing.

Over several months my foot drop improved significantly. That year I entered my first race since college, a 5-mile event. I don't remember how many people were ahead of me (far more than were behind me), but it was a great personal victory. The next year I ran a 10-mile race. The following year I ran a 20-mile race and 2 years later completed my first marathon of 26.2 miles. Since then I have run many marathons and logged thousands of miles running and thousands more on an old Schwinn bicycle. I can nearly run a marathon now without foot drop, but there is always enough foot drop at the end of the run to remind me of the blessing of healing and the answer to prayer.

Do I believe prayer can improve one's health? I am living, running proof of it. I am not alone. Even the medical community is responding to the fact that the majority of Americans say prayer is an important part of their lives. They believe miracles are performed by the power of God. They are sometimes conscious of the presence of God. As a result, spirituality is recognized by many health-care professionals as an important medical tool when developing therapeutic regimens.

This recent interest in prayer and healing has spawned a new term: "complementary medicine." According to Larry Buck of Duke University, complementary medicine seeks to combine prayer and traditional medical practice rather than pit the two against each other. Probably as many as a third of the medical schools in this country have developed courses in alternative/complementary medicine. Most of these emphasize spiritual issues including prayer, religious beliefs, and behavior.

"Statistically, God is good for you," reports David B. Larson of the National Institute of Health Care Research in Rockville, Maryland. Science and religion are no longer enemies—they both require faith.

We are not setting a trap to catch God in;
we are opening a window to watch God work.
—Larry Dossey
Prayer Is Good Medicine

How do we feel about scientific research and prayer? Is God being put to the test? Is our faith in prayer being statistically analyzed? The vast majority of us pray, and we believe our prayers are answered. We aren't holding our breath in anticipation of the results of the next double-blind laboratory study on prayer. We feel that we already have evidence for prayer in our lives, and our lives are the most important laboratories of all.

Medical doctor Randolph Byrd in the *Journal of Christian Nursing*
documented the results of intercessory prayer and healing in his study
of 393 patients randomized upon admission to a coronary care unit.
The first group received intercessory prayer by a group of "born-
again" Christians praying outside the hospital by first name and diagnosis only. The second group did not receive prayers. Updates were
made to the intercessory pray-ers of the prayer group for specific requests, such as "Arthur's diuretic therapy" or "Bill's sleeplessness."
The results published showed that in 21 of 26 categories monitored,
the prayer group showed more improvement.

The *Journal of the American Medical Association* reported on the
first conference on spiritual dimensions in clinical research. The agenda concentrated on three general areas: alcohol and other drug abuses,
mental health, and physical health. The results of the studies reported
at the conference are intriguing:

◆ Religious practices such as prayer, meditation, and reading the
Bible were a way for many people to deal with depression.

◆ Despite chronic disabling disorders such as heart disease and
diabetes, people are less likely to become depressed if they score
high in religious coping (use of religion to adapt to stress). The
more religious behavior, the less the depression.

◆ There is increasing evidence that attention to patients' religious
beliefs and experiences can enhance physical healing and a feeling of general well-being in patients.

◆ The implications of many current studies are that religious beliefs and experiences are an important aspect of hospitaliza-
tions, patients, and their lives. The "healthfulness of prayer"
scale was issued to 100 subjects one day before heart surgery.
Ninety-six of them indicated that prayer was used as a coping
mechanism in dealing with the stress of cardiac surgery. Seven-
ty of them gave it the highest possible rating. These findings
suggest that prayer is perceived as a helpful, direct-action coping mechanism and warrants support by health personnel.

◆ Prayer is a popular and effective way to cope with many life
stressors, including musculoskeletal pain and the stress before
heart surgery. When other coping efforts and remedies have
proven insufficient, people turn to prayer.

◆ Prayer has resulted in decreased intensity of pain in a group of patients with low back pain.

◆ Prayer has resulted in increased hardiness in patients with AIDS or AIDS-related complexes, according to the May 1995 issue of the *Journal of the American Medical Association.*

Other recent studies conclude that

◆ prayer produces much more than a placebo effect;

◆ prayers from a distance are just as effective as prayers up close. The laying on of hands and long-distance prayers are equally effective, according to a study reported by Dossey in *Prayer Is Good Medicine.*

Clearly, the Bible tells us to pray for the health of ourselves and others. James 5:15 asserts that "the prayer offered in faith will make the sick person well." But the primary goal of prayer is not to improve health. "Prayer is an act of self-dedication rather than self-seeking," writes Thomas Merton in *Devotional Classics* (edited by Richard J. Foster and James Smith). "Prayer is not a way to manipulate and coerce God. Rather, prayer is the opening of our heart and mind to a loving God . . . where we create an open, empty space in our hearts for God to work."

We do not need empirical research to convince us that prayer works; two millennia of Church history has proven that.

Interestingly, "medical illness is often a trigger-point for faith," writes Gary Thomas in the January 6, 1997, issue of *Christianity Today.* "A diagnosis of cancer has started many patients on a spiritual journey. Benjamin Carson, pediatric neurosurgeon at Johns Hopkins University, often assigns 'prayer homework' to parents whose children are about to undergo risky brain surgery."

Prayer activates psychological mechanisms such as meaning and hope, according to Michael E. McCullough, writing in the 1995 issue of the *Journal of Psychology and Theology.* It facilitates relaxation, leads to decreased heart rate, lessened muscle tension, and slowed breathing. It can improve our mood and give us an inward sense of peace and calm that extends into other areas of our life.

Nearly 2,000 years ago, Paul observed the connection between our prayer life and our state of mind. "Be anxious for nothing, but in everything by prayer and supplication, with thanksgiving, let your requests be made known to God; and the *peace* of God, which surpasses all understanding, will guard your hearts and minds through Christ Jesus" (Phil. 4:6-7, NKJV, emphasis added).

Despite our prayers, God sometimes does not grant our requests for physical healing in this life. When this happens, the community of faith has a responsibility to provide help. And when nothing but death will take away an illness, patient and family desperately need the support of other believers. In these times, prayer and God's presence will carry us through the dark, discouraging days as we await the ultimate healing of a better tomorrow. Regardless of the outcome, we pray with Julian of Norwich, *O God, by Your goodness give me yourself, for You are enough for me.*

DOCTOR'S ORDERS: RX FOR PRAYER

▶ Pray often.

▶ Pray for the health of your body, mind, emotion, spirit.

▶ Pray for the health of others.

▶ Pray for personal peace, family peace, and world peace.

▶ Talk about prayer.

▶ Read about prayer in books, poems, and songs.

▶ Join a church that prays.

▶ Become involved in the prayer life of your church.

▶ When you're sure, pray. When you doubt, pray.

▶ *Pray.*

He who has a "why" to live for can bear almost any "how."
—Quoted by Frankl from Nietzsche

CHAPTER 6

A WORD FROM THE PROFESSOR . . .
MEANING

ate one Saturday afternoon I lamented to Barbara, "My three hobbies cannot coexist. I can't be a bicyclist, a gardener, and a scholar at the same time." I was frustrated because each of these three activities are time-intensive, high-maintenance endeavors. And even though I enjoy them, the larger question is, "Do these legitimate, healthful, and easily accessible activities fit into the goals and purposes of my life?" All of us face the difficult task of trying to balance our time, resources, and emotional energy. How do we determine the proper mix of vocational, avocational, leisure, family, and social activities in order to discover and enjoy a life of meaning?

At times some of us have asked, "Does my life matter at all?" The writer of Ecclesiastes wondered. "Meaningless! Meaningless!" he cried. "Utterly meaningless! Everything is meaningless" (Eccles. 1:2).

In the same mood, another observed that his life's meaning may be measured by the fact that he had "managed to eat and had escaped being eaten." Is there more to life?

SWINE AND SAINTS

Viktor Frankl hammered out his theories for counseling while he was a prisoner in Auschwitz, Poland, and other concentration camps during World War II. His book *Man's Search for Meaning* is one of my prized possessions. Every year or two I spend time reviewing this small book, which is both autobiographical and theoretical. In it Frankl recounts details of his imprisonment and his attempts to draw meaning out of the horror. At one point, Frankl chides Sigmund Freud for Freud's badly mistaken understanding of "human nature." He quotes Freud: "Let one attempt to expose a number of the most diverse people uniformly to hunger. With the increase of the imperative urge to hunger all individual differences will blur, and in their stead will appear the uniform expression of the one unstilled urge." Frankl's retort is:

> Thank heaven, Sigmund Freud was spared knowing the concentration camps from the inside. His subjects lay on a couch designed in the plush style of Victorian culture, not in the filth of Auschwitz. There, the "individual differences" did not "blur" but, on the contrary, people became more different; people unmasked themselves, both the swine and the saints. And today you need no longer hesitate to use the word "saints."

FINDING MEANING ON THE OTHER SIDE OF DESPAIR

Throughout our lives the thousands of persons we encounter who endure "undeserved suffering" become our teachers. From these "saints" we learn that some things about ourselves, others, and the nature of the universe are understood only after we experience despair.

From 1981 through 1985 I took many late-night walks, arguing with God about my role as a parent of teenagers. Down deep in my gut I knew that Barb and I would survive and so would our children, but the long dark siege of despair took its toll. I cannot dispute, though, the lessons I learned about parenting, faith, intercessory prayer, and my own vulnerability during those years. In the process, my acceptance of and appreciation for others changed, and I found confidence in the ever-present God.

Someone described modern America as a society populated with people who have enough to live on but nothing to live for. We have the means but no meaning. How do we answer the basic questions, "Why am I here?" "What purpose guides my life?"

FINDING MEANING THROUGH OUR SUFFERINGS

A few years ago a friend of mine was fired from a position that involved a lot of organizational politics. Many interested "publics" within the organization claimed an investment in how well his job was done. My friend was hurt by the decision to release him. He felt he had been treated unfairly. I agreed.

In the aftermath, he found himself dealing with anger, damaged self-esteem, bruised pride, and thoughts of retaliation. The only tool I had with which to assist him in his necessary repair work was my presence. Once each week we met for an early morning jog along the shores of Lake Lowell, near Nampa, Idaho.

As we ran, walked, and dodged rabbits, our friendship provided opportunity to address the bitter or better choice. We talked about his choice as a victim of undeserved suffering. He could choose to become bitter and thus shrivel into a small puny creature overcome by his circumstances. Or he could choose to grow from the unfairness of his undeserved suffering and become a better person.

There is no doubt that some people discover meaning without suffering. But most people suffer, and the good news is that in the midst of suffering we can find meaning. Viktor Frankl noted that his chances for survival in the concentration camp were only 1 out of 28. When he entered the camp, he carried with him a manuscript of his first book on counseling. It was taken from him and destroyed. In his book *Man's Search for Meaning*, he lamented that in those early days "it seemed as nothing and no one would survive me; neither a physical or mental child of my own! So I found myself confronted with the question whether under such circumstance my life was ultimately void of any meaning."

Frankl continues:

> A bit later, I remember it seemed to me that I would die in the near future. In this critical situation, however, my concern was different from that of most of my comrades. Their question was, "Will we survive the camp? For, if not, all this suffering has no meaning." The question which beset me was, "Has all this suffering, this dying around us, a meaning? For, if not, ultimately there is no meaning to survival; *for a life whose meaning depends upon such a happenstance—as whether one escapes or not—ultimately would not be worth living at all"* [emphasis added].

FINDING MEANING IN WHAT WE DO

When we are introduced to someone, usually one of the first things we discover is what the person does for a living. I am a student, a teacher, an accountant, a plumber, a sales clerk, or so on, we say. In our society we regard what we do as an important window into who we are.

If you come to my house for dinner, before you leave I will contrive some way to show you my garden, my bicycle, or both. When I come to your house, I'll find myself touring your shop, admiring your paintings, or thumbing through your stamp collection.

Often I hear students say, "Becoming a teacher (social worker, nurse, pastor, or so on) is a way I can fulfill what God wants me to be." Notice the synonymous use of "be" and "do"—our deeds become a source of meaning for us.

FINDING MEANING IN WHAT WE EXPERIENCE

One of the most profound experiences of my entire life occurred July 2, 1990. We were a couple of weeks into a tour of several European countries. That evening, we were in the Pest section of Budapest. The entry in my travel diary for July 2 reads,

> What a profoundly meaningful day! The zenith point of the day came with the Szmfonikus Koncert (Symphony Concert) by the Pesti Community Orchestra and Choir. They performed two pieces—one each by Schumann and Beethoven. . . .
>
> The orchestra, choir, and soloists took us to the heights of ecstasy as they presented Beethoven's Ninth Symphony. The music and lyrics of the potent hymn "Joyful, Joyful, We Adore Thee" were almost more than my capacity for joy could accommodate. . . .
>
> The orchestra members seemed to be folks just like us Americans. They were intent on performing well. They visited and laughed with each other between numbers. They seemed to enjoy the uproarious applause that continued long after they finished playing. The humidity of the city, the poverty of the nation, and the domination of a single political party has not removed the music from the soul of these people. Indeed, God gives a song!

My zest for life heightens dramatically every time I recall that evening. That evening was a wonderful "aha" experience for me. It confirmed the spiritual nature of human existence and the faithful presence of a God who continually invites us into fellowship.

Experiences that connect us with beauty, potential, dreams, God, our spirituality, and others help us discover meaning. In addition to the Budapest concert, I have found meaning in a whole collection of events and relationships—so may all of us. To some extent, we are a composite of a dynamic mix of the places we have been, the folks we have known, the interactions we have shared, and the ongoing memory of the folks, places, and interactions. Again, Frankl's words:

> [A] way of finding meaning in life is by experiencing something—such as goodness, truth, and beauty—by experiencing nature and culture or, last but not least, by experiencing another human being in his very uniqueness—by loving him.

FINDING MEANING THROUGH SERVANTHOOD

Quarrier's Village is located in Scotland 16 miles from the center of Glasgow. This place, sometimes referred to as a children's city of 40 acres and nearly 100 buildings, stands as an ongoing monument in honor of William Quarrier (1829-1903). Born into grinding poverty, Quarrier began working 12 hours a day for six days a week in a pin factory when he was 7 years old. His mother, knowing he had to learn a proper trade, apprenticed him out at 8 years of age to learn shoe-making and shoe repair. By age 14 he was a journeyman shoemaker. By his early 20s he had developed a thriving business and operated multiple shops around Glasgow.

On a cold, raw night in 1864, Quarrier's career path altered dramatically. At the Old Bridge on Jamaica Street, he heard a little street urchin boy cry. He stopped, inquired, and learned that an older orphan boy had stolen all the stock and money of the young match seller. This incident activated Quarrier's growing interest in helping the city's poor children. Years later he wrote about that evening's encounter: "Like Moses of old, I had a strong desire to go down to my brethren, the children of the streets, and endeavor to lead them from a life of misery and shame to one of usefulness and honor" (Magnusson, 1984).

Quarrier organized the homeless children into brigades for shining shoes, selling papers, and delivering parcels. In exchange, they were offered a place to live, received the attention of Christian house parents, acquired education in reading and writing, and had the opportunity to live in an environment of care and support. Additional boys' and girls' homes followed as Quarrier attempted to reach even larger numbers of Glasgow's needy children.

In 1882 Quarrier discontinued the last of his own shoemaking operations in order to give full time to his ministry of assisting children. He announced his intentions by stating, "I believe God will supply, so have decided to depend on him in the time to come for all that I require for myself and my family." Within four years the first buildings at Quarrier's Village began to appear. For more than a century, thousands upon thousands of children have been rescued from their misery to find a place of belonging, safety, education, Christian instruction, medical care, vocational training, and encouragement to live a life of usefulness and honor.

The major roads running through Quarrier's Village are named Faith, Hope, and Love. The Village itself became a warm home of Christian care and development for each new youngster. A phrase that sometimes appeared on Quarrier's printed materials was "Attempt great things for God: Expect great things from God." Quarrier died in 1903 and was buried in the village next to Mount Zion Church. His tombstone's inscription reads, "Entered into rest October 16, 1903, aged 74, William Quarrier, friend of the poor and needy, and founder of the Orphan Homes of Scotland."

Today if you visit Quarrier's Village along the Bridge of Weir, you will find a diversified array of social services for a wide range of Scotland's needy. There are high-quality services for the medically vulnerable, the elderly, epilepsy patients, special-needs children, severely handicapped, and group foster-care provisions, to mention only the major programs.

Quarrier's story illustrates that many persons are not motivated by power or by pleasure, but by service. They live in order to invest themselves in behalf of others. Such persons do not experience inner emptiness; rather, they are fulfilled with a sense of worthwhileness.

Selfless servanthood brings our attention to Jesus Christ. Paul wrote:

Do nothing out of selfish ambition or vain conceit, but in humility consider others better than yourselves. Each of you should look not only to his own interests, but also to the interests of others. Your attitude should be the same as that of Christ Jesus:

Who . . . [took] the very nature of a servant *(Phil. 2:3-7).*

Mark preserved Jesus' own words regarding this theme:

Whoever wants to become great among you must be your servant, and whoever wants to be first must be slave of all. For even the Son of Man did not come to be served, but to serve, and give his life as a ransom for many *(Mark 10:43-45).*

WHOLENESS, FULLNESS, AND MEANING

Spirituality is the integrating core for wholeness. We may be *empty people with full schedules.* We may complain about too-full schedules, too-full days, too many meetings, too many expectations, too few hours in the day, and too many demands for time and attention. If this is the case, our goal should be to become *full people with meaningful schedules (lives).*

Each of us must determine a central purpose, mission, or core around which all of life is organized. This does not mean that we will be free to sit and sip iced tea two hours each day without any obligations. In fact, we will continue to be busy. The difference is that we will allow our faith in God to be the organizing principle of our lives. We will view all of life through an empty tomb and seek the Lordship of the risen and living Christ over all areas of our lives—including our calendars.

Wholeness means that the totality of our lives rotates around this center of faith. Out of this God-indwelt center flow life's choices, intentions, relationships, and goals. Jesus spoke of this singularity of a full and meaningful life when He summarized all the commandments as follows:

"Hear, O Israel, the Lord our God, the Lord is one. Love the Lord your God with all your heart and with all your soul and with all your mind and with all your strength." The second is this: "Love your neighbor as yourself." There is no commandment greater than these *(Mark 12:29-31).*

A Christian seeks God in every dimension of existence. He gives our lives meaning. College chaplain Gene Schandorff states the issue plainly: "We all have as much of God as we now desire—because God desires that we have as much of Him as we will receive."

THE PROF'S HOMEWORK ASSIGNMENT:
OWNING A SAINT'S PRAYER

For a Christian the purpose of life may be reduced to a single word. Although it is too simplistic for most contexts, the single word is *Jesus.* A prayer of St. Patrick shows that for a Christian, *meaning* means Jesus. Read/pray aloud the following prayer. Before the day is over, read it aloud to at least one other person.

I arise today through God's strength to pilot me,
God's might to uphold me, God's wisdom to guide me,
God's eye to look before me, God's ear to hear for me,
God's word to speak for me, God's hand to guard me,
God's way to lie before me, God's shield to protect me.
Christ be with me, Christ before me, Christ behind me, Christ in me,
Christ beneath me, Christ above me, Christ on my right, Christ on my left,
Christ when I lie down, Christ when I sit down, Christ when I arise,
Christ in the heart of everyone who thinks of me,
Christ in the mouth of everyone who speaks of me,
Christ in every eye that sees me, Christ in every ear that hears me.

—a benediction by St. Patrick

It is not very often things they need. What they need much more is what we offer them. In these twenty years of work amongst the people, I have come more and more to realize that it is being unwanted that is the worst disease that any human can ever experience. Nowadays we have found medicine for TB [tuberculosis], and consumption can be cured. For all kinds of diseases there are medicines and cures. But for being unwanted, except there are willing hands to serve and there's a loving heart to love, I don't think this terrible disease can ever be cured.

—Mother Teresa

CHAPTER 7

A WORD FROM THE PROFESSOR . . .
RELATIONSHIPS

MEET PASTOR BOB

Bob Morris, preacher, farmer, and teacher, represents a large host of people who marked my life. He served as pastor of the Ontario Heights Friends Church in Ontario, Oregon, which was a simple basement building on a gravel road. The cement floor and walls of the small sanctuary enclosed the pine slat pews and the central heat system, a kerosene stove. The bathroom was reached easily by a path out back, except when the snow and ice interfered.

Bob Morris hired out to the farmers to supplement what must have been a poverty-level salary. I enjoyed the days he worked alongside us on our farm and shared noon meals at our table. Bob's major influence on my life, however, came through his role as leader of the Ontario Heights 4-H Club. He took seriously the development of the boys who showed up for meetings. He worked on the *H* themes of Hands, Head, Heart, and Health. In addition, he modeled what it meant to be an honest, helpful, hopeful, humble man. He taught us how to grow crops, raise cattle, judge cattle, show cattle in competition, tie a multiplicity of knots, and a variety of other skills relevant for farm boys. But mostly I learned about life and Christian character from this man. Bob painted creatively, lovingly, and winsomely on the canvas of my life.

Over the years, thousands of other persons—childhood buddies, Sunday School teachers, coaches, neighbors, members of our extended family—have taken their turn with the paintbrush. New strokes continue to be added. Now they are from colleagues, supervisors, children, grandchildren, men in the prayer group, and professional contacts.

Some of the designs I recognize; others are more subtle and have gone unnoticed. Without a doubt, we are social beings, interdependent on one another. Like it or not, we are enmeshed deeply within the social, political, economic exchange structures of our society.

QUALITY CONTROL—QC

This is a QC—quality control—chapter on relationships. What ensures that our relationships are healthy, growing, and Christian? QC issues often reduce to simple matters, such as time. Paul Taylor, staff writer for the *Washington Post*, examined "time deficit families" who are engaged in marathon juggling acts. In his report, which ran January 14-20, 1991, Taylor quoted social historian Barbara Defoe Whitehead: "When a shoe is lost, a cold car engine fails to turn over, or the baby fills his diaper just after he's been zipped into his snowsuit, or the staff meeting runs late, the whole intricate schedule can unravel and fall apart." None of us are surprised when we read that research documents the fact that parents spend considerably less time with their children now than parents did 30 years ago.

Wholeness in relationships involves time but much more. It is multidimensional. Wholeness requires a healthy relationship with God, oneself, other people, the environment. Life does not happen within a vacuum or a sterile laboratory. Life unfolds in the context of a given time, in a given place, occupied by a specific mix of people with particular religious, cultural, class, and traditional characteristics.

TREAT OTHERS AS YOU WISH TO BE TREATED

Treating others as one wishes to be treated is the beginning point for marriage partners, business partners, tennis partners, and all other partnerships linking us with others. New Testament physician Luke preserved Jesus' Golden Rule for human relationships with these words: "Just as you want men to do to you, you also do to them likewise" (Luke 6:31, NKJV). This Golden Rule of respect declares that I value you as an equal with me and therefore will treat you as I wish to be treated. Luke cited the mercy of our Heavenly Father as the model we must follow with all people, even those who may misuse us. He quoted Jesus: "Be merciful, just as your Father also is merciful" (Luke 6:36, NKJV).

The principle brings to mind the "law of reciprocity." As a child I sometimes heard my mother make comments such as "I owe Nellie a letter," or "I owe the Stewarts a dinner." Reciprocity serves as a pragmatic and practical guide for human interaction. Reciprocity is a way by which much gets done in society. My farmer dad traded work and farm machinery with his neighbors. The golden rule of human relationships, however, implies more than "I'll scratch your back if you'll scratch mine."

"The law of mutuality" is a principle that declares there is more than keeping score or counting who has done what, when, how often, and whether it is fair in comparison with what I have done. Mutuality reinforces my goal to treat all persons with respect and fairness. Mutuality calls us to engage in the give-and-take of social exchanges with purposeful effort. Someone referred to this as "having as much sense as a goose." The V formation used by geese adds a greater flying range for the flock than if each goose flies alone. The single goose quickly returns to the formation with the flock when it recognizes the additional thrust that comes from alignment with others. We can go farther, faster, and easier by going together.

Paul emphasized the advantages of living by the V formation of the Golden Rule. The apostle used the relationship that exists among the many parts of the body to reveal the vital force of mutuality. The human body has many separate parts but forms a single unit. In fact, a disconnected ear, foot, or liver has no value separated from the whole. Apart from connection with the whole body, each separate part will die and decay.

> Now indeed there are many members, yet one body. And the eye cannot say to the hand, "I have no need of you"; nor again the head to the feet, "I have no need of you." No, much rather, those members of the body which seem to be weaker are necessary. . . . there should be no schism in the body, but . . . the members should have the same care for one another. And if one suffers, all the members suffer with it; or if one member is honored, all the members rejoice with it *(1 Cor. 12:20-22, 25-26, NKJV)*.

LOVE OTHERS AS YOURSELF

A second dimension of wholeness in relationships, loving others as oneself, extends beyond reciprocity and mutuality. The word *love* is bigger than afternoon television soaps and late-night X-rated movies. *Love* references a divine-like quality. George Lyons in *Holiness in Everyday Life* captures well a higher order of love: "Love is humility, gentleness, patience, and tolerance in action. Love is not primarily a feeling, nor even a disposition; it is *active goodwill, seeking what is in the long-term best interest of the other*" (emphasis added).

Love is not some fuzzy abstract concept for stuffy theological debates. Rather, love is intentional good will seeking the other's best in specific plans and actions. Many fuss and fume these days about the perceived extremes of political correctness. But there seems to be a similar movement among many Christians that may be called evangelical correctness. This movement would force everyone to think and speak with the "right" words and phrases. In addition, this perspective would require everyone to belong to the "correct" political party and organizations. Genuine Christian love, however, is not simply thinking and speaking correctly, although orthodoxy is an important issue. Genuine Christian love is *acting right*.

A confusion between "thinking right" and "acting right" can lead to tragic consequences. I know a sincere young couple, recently converted and learning well what obedience to Christ means, who believes they must firmly support all elements of "evangelical correctness" pumped out by local Christian radio stations. Their belligerent attitudes and win-the-theological-argument-regardless-of-the-necessary-rancor-required mind-set is tearing their extended family apart. Their non-Christian family members find the couple less Christian in actions than they were before they confessed Jesus as Lord. In a recent family squabble over homosexuality, every trace of love was lost in the overriding goal of winning the argument with "evangelical correctness." There is never an argument (or a policy, election, or social institution) important enough to set aside acting Christlike. Thinking and speaking in "approved" Christian phrases and categories never replaces representing Christ in our actions.

WHAT A JESUS WE HAVE IN A FRIEND

Martin E. Marty, church historian, in the October 1981 issue of *HIS* magazine, describes Christian love in concrete actions with a crisp play on words when he says, "What a Jesus we have in a friend." Many of us have been strengthened and given courage to carry on when simply hearing the words of Joseph M. Scriven's hymn:

> *What a Friend we have in Jesus,*
> *All our sins and griefs to bear!*
> *What a privilege to carry*
> *Ev'rything to God in prayer!*

Jesus indeed is our Friend. But Marty says we see genuine Christian love at its best when Jesus comes to us in the person of a friend. To be Christ to a friend does not mean that we join the Godhead or assume divine perfection. Joan Wulff suggests, "The Biblical witness is sufficiently clear: Divine character is somehow to flow through fallible humans, even though they do not thenceforth become perfect. . . . It is not nonsensical to say 'What a Jesus we have in a friend;' it may better protect the character of sacrificial love than to sing, 'What a Friend we have in Jesus.'"

"NEIGHBOR" IS A VERB

The challenge to love others as we love ourselves is found in Jesus' summary of the great commandments. "'You shall love the LORD your God with all your heart, with all your soul, with all your strength, and with all your mind,' and 'your neighbor as yourself'" (Luke 10:27, NKJV). The context in which this commandment is discussed is in relationship to the story of the good Samaritan. The good Samaritan, although from a despised category of persons himself, invested time, gave money, inconvenienced himself, and made arrangements for the continued care of the injured. No smooth-talking Christianity implied here. Rather, actions. Christians change the word "neighbor" from a noun to a verb. In essence, Jesus said we must *neighbor* those experiencing needs. That is, we must take actions to meet the needs of others.

Jesus' premise that we love ourselves is foundational. Stated simply, I can't love you until I love myself. Wholeness in our relationships with others is contingent upon how well we relate to the person in the mirror. I cannot achieve wholeness until I accept, value, and love myself. This proper acceptance of self becomes the springboard, then, for me to accept, value, and love you as a person.

GIVING MYSELF FOR THE WELL-BEING OF OTHERS

Meaningful relationships demand hard work and persistence—sometimes a lifetime. When Albrecht Dürer (1471-1528) was a poor young artist, another young aspiring artist agreed to do manual labor in order to earn a living for the two of them. This arrangement allowed Dürer to study and paint. It was planned that later the friend would take his turn to study and become a painter.

By the time Dürer gained success as a painter, his friend's hands had become twisted and stiff and no longer capable of creating art. Dürer could do nothing to restore the hands of his friend. He did, however, paint his friend's hands while they were clasped in prayer. One of Dürer's most famous paintings, "Hands Folded in Prayer," preserves the story of the high price required for relationships.

HAVING THE SAME ATTITUDE AS CHRIST

Sometimes relationships demand so much that we are left empty. Phil. 2:1-11 reports how Jesus emptied himself in behalf of others. He gave up all that He had, not holding on to His eternal glory. Rather, "[He] made himself nothing, taking the very nature of a servant, being made in human likeness. And being found in appearance as a man, he humbled himself and became obedient to death—even death on a cross!" (Phil. 2:7-8).

Let's not be too eager to dismiss this scripture with "Well, that's a God thing." Although we expect God to make a supreme sacrifice in behalf of His children, this passage has our names written on it. Paul writes earlier in the same chapter,

> Do nothing out of selfish ambition or vain conceit, but in humility consider others better than yourselves. Each of you should look not only to your own interests, but also to the interests of others. *Your attitude should be the same as that of Christ Jesus:*
> Who, being in very nature God,
> did not consider equality with God something to be grasped,
> but made himself nothing *(Phil. 2:3-7, emphasis added).*

This emptying myself, then, is as much about me as it is Jesus Christ.

SPIRITUAL DISCIPLINE OR CODEPENDENCY

We often discuss the "disease" identified as codependency. Considerable debate exists among addictions professionals as to whether it is appropriate to declare codependency as a disease. I contend that codependency is as much an addiction as alcohol, tobacco, gambling, shopping, work, and exercise. Several key factors characterize the maladaptive lifestyle of codependency. Codependents

1. are interested in managing or controlling the behaviors of others;
2. accept responsibility and/or guilt for what others do;
3. focus on what goes on outside themselves, especially in the lives of those they wish to control.

A codependent, then, will make almost any sacrifice of his or her schedule and resources in order to achieve goals in the behaviors of some other person or persons.

CAREGIVING FOR OTHERS

How does codependency differ from acceptable spiritual care? Sometimes we blur the distinction between healthy sacrificial love in behalf of others, which flows out of our commitment to Christ, with codependency. Conservative parents and pastors are especially at risk of falling into codependency. Ask yourself these questions:

How do I try to control the behaviors of some (for example, late adolescent and adult children, or church leaders)?

How do I assume responsibility for what some do or don't do?

To what extent do I ignore dealing with what is going on inside of me because I am deeply engaged in what is going on in the lives of others?

Significant implications flow from the way we answer the above questions. Wholeness and balance characterize healthy spiritual disciplines. In contrast, the codependent is obsessed or consumed with the control of another and the accepting of responsibility for the other's actions. Thus, the codependent rarely addresses his or her own needs and goals. The one serving Christ by serving others is committed to a complete and full life. Service to others is important but is only one segment of the person's life. Further, one's social life does not rotate around only the addicted or problem-plagued person. A variety of social activities with many other persons engage the Christian service-giver of wholeness. In addition, the person of wholeness is engaged in the development of the total self—body, mind, and spirit.

COMMITTED CONNECTION WITH OTHERS

Mike Yaconelli in the April-May 1980 issue of *Wittenburg Door* describes Christians who lack commitment to one another as "religious billiard balls." By this designation he suggests that we bump into each other but have no connection with one another—relationships that aren't relationships. "We have opted," Yaconelli suggests, "for slick, strobe-lighted, lip-gloss Christianity in place of dirty, risky, tear-stained long-term relationships. We have allowed others to become images rather than friends, people we know rather than people we love."

Yaconelli helps us recall the example of Jesus who challenged us to love genuinely—not simply with bumper stickers and cute sayings on the church's bulletin board. Jesus commanded, "Love one another as I have loved you. Greater love has no one than this, than to lay down one's life for his friends" (John 15:12-13, NKJV). John emphasized further the high demands of a love relationship: "By this we know love, because He laid down His life for us. And we also ought to lay down our lives for the brethren" (1 John 3:16, NKJV).

John's suggestion that we "lay down our lives" describes the contract we enter into as Christians. He goes on to spell out the fine print of our commitment: "But whosoever has this world's goods, and sees his brother in need, and shuts up his heart from him, how does the love of God abide in him? My little children, let us not love [only] in word or in tongue, but in deed and in truth" (1 John 3:17-18, NKJV).

Take note, Christian. How's your love life? Are you holding up your end of the contract?

THE PROF'S HOMEWORK ASSIGNMENT: BELONGING

Do all our family members know that they belong simply because they exist? Or have we established conditions for belonging? Have we made someone's acceptance contingent upon his or her performance? And besides, who decided what is the right standard of performance? Are we able to say, "I will always love you and accept you regardless"? We may have some repair work to do if we cannot say this or choose not to endorse this attitude. This matter of "acceptance if" instead of "acceptance regardless" deserves both thoughtful prayer and discussion with a mature Christian mentor or counselor.

One of the brethren had been insulted by another and he wanted to take revenge. He came to Abbot Silos and told him what had taken place, saying: I am going to get even, Father. But the elder besought him to leave the affair in the hands of God. No, said the brother, I will not give up until I have made that fellow pay for what he said. Then the elder stood up and began to pray in these terms: O God, Thou art no longer necessary to us, and we no longer need Thee to take care of us since, as this brother says, we both can and will avenge ourselves. At this the brother promised to give up his idea of revenge.

—Thomas Merton
The Wisdom of the Desert

CHAPTER 8

A WORD FROM THE PROFESSOR . . .
FORGIVENESS

Yonkers, New York, police officers arrested David Berkowitz, a postal worker, former auxiliary policeman, and confessed "Son of Sam" killer. Shortly after Berkowitz confessed to the six murders, his father, Nathan Berkowitz, met with news reporters. The elder Berkowitz stated, "If David did these things, I don't expect you parents to forgive him. That would be too much to ask of you."

He continued: "My loss is not because of a son whom I adopted, but my loss is multiplied by what each and every one of the parents of these crime victims feels in his or her heart."

78

Is forgiveness ever too much to ask? Are some actions unforgivable? Are some persons too base and degraded to forgive? And what difference would it make if the parents of Berkowitz's victims extended forgiveness?

Does offered forgiveness change anything? Yes! It changes persons and situations. *Forgiveness* is a multidimensional word. It points upward, inward, and outward. It ushers us simultaneously into the study of theology, mental health, and sociology.

I met Greg 20 years ago while I was a social worker at the Nashville Workhouse. Convicted male criminals with sentences of less than 11 months and 29 days were assigned to this medium-security facility. Greg taught me many things about retaliation. He showed me how desperately we all need to forgive and be forgiven. He put in his time but experienced no rehabilitation. Less than one year after entering the Nashville Workhouse, he returned to the streets of Nashville as a man eager and prepared to "get even" with every witness and legal functionary who had helped place him in jail. His most novel (and probably most expensive) plan was to hire a cement company to fill with concrete the basement of a key witness who testified against him. Greg spent his time in jail refusing to accept responsibility and planning how to make people pay.

Greg needed to hear the strong multidimensional word *forgiveness*. Forgiveness could have opened doors that would have contributed to his rehabilitation. Forgiveness opens the door to fellowship with God. Forgiveness opens the door to healthy self-acceptance and emotional well-being. Forgiveness opens the door to restored relationships with others. It is a three-dimensional concept:

Forgiveness is a God-and-me word.

Forgiveness is an I-and-me word.

Forgiveness is a you-and-me word.

FORGIVENESS IS A GOD-AND-ME WORD

Our class of seventh grade boys were playing catch during the lunch hour. My friend Reed threw me a hard fast one. It stung the hand that had not caught a baseball all winter. Reed teased, "What's the matter, Jerry? Did that pitch hurt?"

"No way," I snarled back. "That didn't hurt."

A deep pain jabbed my heart. I wasn't tough. Not at all. I was a liar. And the visiting evangelist who passed through our town had taught me well where liars were sure to go. I told a lie to my boyhood friend, but my sin was against God. Deep in my young heart I sensed failure. I felt shame for lying about such a silly little matter.

Centuries before, a powerful king walked on the roof of his palace. In the yard of a nearby house he saw a beautiful woman bathing. The king exploited his power and called her to the palace, where he engaged in sexual relations with her. She became pregnant. The king maneuvered circumstances to have her husband killed so he could take the woman as his wife.

Then and now God holds us accountable. A moral law of the universe is understood well in the simple phrase "Your sin will find you out" (Num. 32:23). A faithful prophet pointed his bony finger under the king's nose and declared, "You despicable man. You defiled a woman, murdered her husband, and failed the nation. More importantly, you sinned against God Almighty and do not deserve His mercy." (See 2 Sam. 11 and 12.)

King David experienced the same sickening self-realization I felt, hundreds of years later, on the south lawn of Ontario Junior High School—a moment of truth in which we admit, "I am a sinner. I have sinned against God." King David declared, "I acknowledge my transgressions, And my sin is ever before me. Against You, You only, have I sinned, And done this evil in Your sight" (Ps. 51:3-4, NKJV).

David's only hope was forgiveness. My only hope was forgiveness. "Wash me thoroughly from my iniquity, And cleanse me from my sin," David prayed. "Create in me a clean heart, O God" (Ps. 51:2, 10, NKJV). David's prayer is my prayer. His sin and mine remind us of two wonderful truths about forgiveness: One, none of us is so good we don't need forgiveness. Two, none of us is so bad we can't be forgiven.

There is something wonderful and powerful about the mercy of God at work when we are forgiven. It is a multifaceted process, involving *remission, reconciliation, relationship,* and *righteousness.*

God's gift of forgiveness is granted to us whenever we repent for what we have done, declare a desire to change our heart, and ask for grace to live the way God wants us to live. Through *remission* God cancels or releases us from the debt of blame and penalty we should face because of our sins. Our sins are barriers or obstacles keeping us from fellowship with God. God, through forgiveness, releases us of the penalties we owe for the sins we have committed. No longer, then, are our sins obstacles between us and God.

Through His gracious forgiveness, God brings us into a state of *reconciliation* with himself. Previously we were separated and at odds with (alienated from) God. But God in Christ Jesus has arranged an agreement between two formerly warring parties.

Christians dare to declare that through forgiveness we enter into a *relationship* with God. In the mystery of God's plan we are brought into a personal relationship with God in Christ. He is closer to us than the closest of friends and relatives. Because of forgiveness we are near to God and feel no separation or barriers between us.

Through our relationship with God we become participants in His *righteousness*. We cannot earn God's approval by works of discipleship, regardless of our effort. Righteousness is an ongoing outcome of our walk with God. Forgiven Christians enjoy fellowship with God and, in the process, begin to become like the One with whom we talk, walk, and share. Righteousness is not a destination point but a journey. Righteousness is a process dependent upon the present and continuous ministry of Christ within us.

FORGIVENESS IS AN I-AND-ME WORD

As I walked across campus to my office, I mumbled to myself, "That's just not like me." I was disappointed because I had become upset over a minor issue in a meeting. My impatience caused me to make a comment that violated one of my basic principles. Now I was wondering why I had reacted as I did.

This incident illustrates how we use "self talk" to converse with ourselves. We view ourselves as objects for evaluation, criticism, and change. "I" evaluate "me." Continuously "I" am making judgments about "me." These judgments lead to positive self-regard or negative self-regard or some midpoint between the two extremes.

We should be our own most honest critics. Too often, though, we move beyond criticism to vicious denunciation. We demand perfectionism but discover mistake-prone mortals staring back when we look in the mirror. We expect ourselves to be poised, wise, witty, self-controlled spiritual dynamos. Instead, we find ourselves to be confused, foolish, dull, self-indulgent losers.

The man I see when I stand in front of the mirror is partly a creation of the messages received from people around me. All of us care how others perceive us. An early American sociologist, Charles Horton Cooley, described the "looking-glass self." Cooley's "looking-glass self" (mirror) model suggests that we respond to others in a series of sequential steps. Consider the first day of the semester when I meet with the social policy class. *Step 1:* I recognize the 45 students in the class are watching me and making an evaluation about my appearance, competence, approachability, and so on. *Step 2:* I determine what I believe they are thinking about me. *Step 3:* I develop a judgment about myself on the basis of what I believe the students are thinking. In other words, I allow them to be my "looking glass" (mirror) to see what I am like.

Much of what I see comes from the mirrors held around me across the years by parents, siblings, friends, teachers, and so on. As we mature, we become more selective about which mirrors we regard as important. We learn to become more skilled in serving as our own most important mirror. And as Christians, we observe intently the mirror held before us by God the Holy Spirit.

I remember the night well. Our trilevel house provided me space for some sturdy soul-searching. Paul's words "What a wretched man I am!" (Rom. 7:24) were the only words I could repeat. For more than an hour I anguished in prayer over attitudes and actions I had permitted in my life. That evening I knew that Paul spoke of me when he said, "For all have sinned and fall short of the glory of God" (Rom. 3:23). As the time passed I was able to hear the instructions of the apostle of love when he promised, "If we confess our sins, he is faithful and just and will forgive us our sins and purify us from all unrighteousness" (1 John 1:9).

Before the end of the second hour of intense self-appraisal, I accepted the assurance "I am forgiven, I am forgiven, I am forgiven." In Christ Jesus we may look in the mirror and find a person washed of all the grime and filth of painful years, experiences, and relationships. As Paul noted, "If anyone is in Christ, he is a new creation; the old has gone, the new has come!" (2 Cor. 5:17; see also Rom. 6:11 and Col. 3:1-3). Through God's forgiveness we rewrite our personal history.

A revision of our personal history does not change the dates, places, actors, actions, words, or attitudes of earlier times. Forgiveness does not erase those acute traumatic experiences or those days and nights of despair. But forgiven persons discover that the meaning of those former days and ways is changed. In Christ Jesus we may reinterpret the meaning of those former events, actions, and relationships. Although we cannot change what we did or what was done to us, we can change our perception of those events. We can redefine the way we permit ourselves to be influenced by those former circumstances.

Recently a 30-year-old acquaintance reported, "I've ruined my life. I'm a terrible person, and I don't have a future." Not so. We serve a God of second chances, fresh starts, and new beginnings. True—we remain accountable for what we have done in the past; we may need to make amends. However, as a forgiven person, each of us can say, "Today is the first day of the rest of my life. If Jesus Christ forgives and accepts me, so may "I" forgive and accept "me." Forgiveness is indeed an I-and-me word.

FORGIVENESS IS A YOU-AND-ME WORD

During the 1996 United States election campaign, Idaho Public Television featured an interview with one of the state's leading politicians. The reporter asked the 25-year veteran of Idaho politics if he could identify any mistakes he had made as an elected official. Without hesitation he replied, "No, I can't recall any mistakes I have made." The reporter rephrased the question to inquire if in retrospect he wished he could redo some things and do them differently. The politician could not think of any areas for possible improvement.

"What planet does this guy live on?" I said aloud to the television. Most of us can create a list from yesterday alone of a half dozen things we did wrong or would do differently if given a second chance.

Political leaders aren't the only persons who need to learn to admit mistakes and apologize. Many problems in business and civic circles could be resolved if we would recommit ourselves to saying we're sorry. And most families in America would benefit from an increased willingness to forgive.

Forgiveness at the horizontal level—forgiveness for each other—is essential to wholeness. Consider four characteristics of forgiveness:

1. Forgiven people forgive.
2. Forgiven people know that forgiving is a precondition for forgiveness.
3. Forgiven people speak plainly.
4. Forgiven people have bad memories.

Forgiven People Forgive

The Associated Press released a human interest story about Michael Carlucci, who spent three years in a Connecticut state prison for a manslaughter conviction. Carlucci allegedly killed Scott Everett in 1987 while both men were under the influence of substances. Less than one month into his imprisonment, Carlucci received a letter from his victim's father, Walter Everett. Rev. Everett informed Carlucci that he had forgiven him through the love of God. Each month thereafter Pastor Everett wrote a letter to Carlucci. Two and one-half years into his prison sentence, Carlucci received Everett as a visitor. They reached out to shake hands but instead spontaneously embraced each other. Everett recalled, "We both started crying." Later Rev. Everett officiated at Carlucci's wedding.

Walter Everett followed Paul's counsel: "Be kind and compassionate to one another, forgiving each other, just as in Christ God forgave you" (Eph. 4:32). The murder of July 26, 1987, changed Rev. Everett's life forever. Never again would he enjoy a conversation with his son. Never would he have the privilege of baptizing his boy's children. The list of missed joys goes on and on. But forgiveness was a choice that he alone could make. He could not wish away the pain. By forgiving Carlucci, Rev. Everett was not pretending that the murder had not occurred. Rather, by forgiving Carlucci, Everett was participating with the divine One. He accepted God's offer of help to restore hope, emotional balance, and sufficient reason for living.

Developmental theorists refer to *fixation*. This happens when we get stuck at some stage in life and fail to process the issues causing us great pain. Emotional and spiritual fixation occurs when I am unwilling to forgive another for something done against me. Two things result. First, I become stuck in the tragedy of the hurtful circumstances. Second, I grant control to the one who wronged me. When we forgive, we create other options for our life. Someone observed correctly, "Forgiveness does not change the past, but it does enlarge the future."

Walter Everett seized his own future when he forgave Michael Car-lucci. Everett's son was still dead. Genuine forgiveness does not ignore, excuse, or deny the injury. But forgiveness gives God permission to cut the chains that bind us to the past and work His miracle of healing within us.

Forgiven People Know That Forgiving Is a Precondition for Forgiveness

The Beatitudes declare, "Blessed are the merciful, for they will be shown mercy" (Matt. 5:7). In the next chapter Matthew spoke directly: "For if you forgive men when they sin against you, your heavenly Father will also forgive you. But if you do not forgive men their sins, your Father will not forgive your sins" (6:14-15).

If this were the text of next Sunday's sermon, just imagine the traffic jam at the vestibule doors as we would rush out to find those we need to forgive. Simply stated, forgiveness of others is necessary if we expect God to forgive us. Recall the familiar phrase in the Lord's Prayer "Forgive us our debts [sins], As we forgive our debtors [those who sin against us]" (Matt. 6:12, NKJV).

Reconciliation with our fellow humans takes precedence over religious ceremony. Making things right with neighbors should be a high priority for us; according to Jesus, "If you bring your gift to the altar, and there remember that your brother has something against you, leave your gift there before the altar, and go your way. First be reconciled to your brother, and then come and offer your gift" (Matt. 5:23-24, NKJV).

Forgiven People Speak Plainly

When is forgiveness not forgiveness? You've probably heard someone say, "OK, I'll forgive you this one time, but never again!" This kind of conditional language is inappropriate when seeking or granting forgiveness. Likewise, there is a world of difference between the following two statements:

I'm sorry that what I said upset you.

I'm sorry for what I said to you.

The first statement allows blame to be placed on the offended party. "After all, if you weren't so thin-skinned, you wouldn't have been offended by what I said," the speaker implies. Blame is pushed off on the offended, even while appearing to be asking for forgiveness.

Forgiving people speak plainly. We owe honesty both to ourselves and to others involved. We may say, "I was hurt deeply by what you

did. I know that the consequences of what you did will be . . . , but God
in Christ has forgiven. I pray that God will grant me the ability to forgive
you completely so both of us may go on without hate and animosity."

Forgiven People Have Bad Memories

Nearly 15 years of service as a dean of students in Christian liberal
arts colleges has allowed me many opportunities for alienating students
(and their families). I never awakened any morning with the intent of
making bad decisions. I must confess, however, that there are some
things I would do differently if repeating the assignment. Sometimes
even my "right" decisions were misunderstood and were a source of
frustration for those involved. I've received angry letters, listened to dis-
gusted callers, heard my name and intentions ridiculed, and, of course,
had my house covered with toilet paper.

The most grievous insult occurred in the mid-1980s. I went to campus early one morning to see graffiti directed at me plastered all over
campus. Some of the comments were vulgar and obscene. All the words
hurt. Student leaders, colleagues, and campus cleaning crews joined together to erase the graffiti. The sessions of reconciliation with the two
perpetrators were some of the most significant moments of forgiving
grace experienced in my entire professional career. This week, more than
a decade later, I noticed the brick wall of one building that had been de-
faced by the two angry students. I thought about the men, now in their
mid-30s, and wondered how they are doing. I rejoice to realize that our
memories can be cleansed of those things that could disable us.

We must be forgivers and forgetters. Someone reminded Clara Bar-
ton, founder of the American Red Cross, of a person who once did a
hurtful thing to her. She remarked, "I distinctly remember forgetting that
incident." We may remember with our heads but by God's grace choose
to forget with our hearts. When we forgive, we move on with today and
anticipate tomorrow with joy.

THE PROF'S HOMEWORK ASSIGNMENT:
DISCARD ALL FORGIVEN IOUs

Let's be honest. Have we forgiven someone but saved an IOU, just in case? Either
forgiveness is complete, total, withholding nothing, or it is not genuine forgiveness. Answer this question: Have I saved back a forgiveness IOU? If so, what
must I do?

We are what we repeatedly do.
Excellence, then, is not an act, but a habit.
                                        —Aristotle

CHAPTER 9

A WORD FROM THE DOCTOR . . .
HABITS

B eing healthy is having confidence in the future," wrote Bob Hoke
in the February 1968 issue of the *Archives of Environmental Health.*
"The healthy man's future does not happen passively to him; it is
an active extension of his life. *For him the future is created by his choices
and decisions.* Instead of the future coming to him, he takes himself to it
and his living becomes a joint creation. Health is a participation in the
creation, a participation in one's own being, a commitment to one's
living in the world. To be healthy is to celebrate one's life."

Roy was a year older than me. In college he and I were members of
the cross-country and track teams, though he was not the stereotypical
athlete. He was slight of build, with a strange stride and poor muscle development. He would enter all the long races, and during his first year
he was usually near the end of the pack. I recall looking down my long,
arrogant nose at Roy because I perceived myself as fast and athletic.

But Roy always seemed to feel part of the team. He cheered everyone else on and never seemed to envy our success or victories. He was
very coachable and worked hard. After track season he didn't stop running—he kept on working, plodding, sweating, and training, and by his
senior year he was placing in the fourth or fifth positions in some races.

He loved the team, he loved to participate, and he obviously loved
his personal improvement. He seemed to have learned and lived the

valuable lesson expressed in George Sheehan's book *Personal Best:* "The honorable thing is not to excel against others but to excel against yourself. . . . The real contest is within. The real trophy is the self . . . our total self—body, mind, and spirit."

Roy realized that the body is the starting point. As stated in Sheehan's book, "In turning to our bodies, we turn to our minds and souls, to the whole that is one's self. . . . The normal life is one of continual expansion. . . . Growth does not occur in [a] haphazard way."

Over the past 40 years Roy has been an inspiration to many. He has maintained a healthful lifestyle. He is an outstanding coach and teacher; a committed, growing Christian; and a devoted father and husband. He is a consummate example of good choices and healthy behavior.

Roy remains trim, strong, enthusiastic, happy, and youthful. He runs races much faster now than I can and has a lot more ribbons than I do.

One thing he does *not* have is a long, arrogant nose.

**The conditions of conquests
are always easy.
We have but to toil awhile,
endure awhile,
believe always, and never turn back.**

—Simms

**Great works are performed not by
strength, but by perseverance.**

—Samuel Johnson

CHICKEN VS. EGG, OR CHARACTER VS. HABITS

Great character obviously results in healthy positive habits, and positive habits can contribute to the development and growth of character. Right behaviors, positive mental attitudes, and a good work ethic can have tremendous benefit but cannot in and of themselves change character. There needs to come a moment, a spiritual experience, that either makes or initiates the making of the true character of our inner selves.

My father-in-law, George Olson, tells about the time his marriage was in jeopardy because of his serious problems with alcohol. One Saturday night during that time in his life George went to a Youth for Christ rally, where he decided to go forward and commit his life to Jesus Christ. As he left the auditorium, he threw away his cigarettes. When he arrived home, he poured out his alcohol supply. He began attending church faithfully. He read and studied his Bible and changed his life to fit its principles. He began a lifelong pursuit of helping the needy, pouring himself into the needs of the down-and-out. He faithfully visited inner-city missions to present his life testimony. He gave food and supplies to the poor and tried to relieve suffering in any way that he could. George's character change preceded his new habits. Yet his changed habits empowered him to give effective, useful, productive service to the world around him.

My good friend Scott, on the other hand, had a serious heart attack at age 32 from severe occlusive coronary artery disease and had to undergo emergency and multiple bypass surgeries. His father had died at age 35 from the same disease, as had many of his male ancestors. Scott was an intelligent, highly motivated business entrepreneur with a lovely wife and two young children. He decided he was not going to die without a fight. From the day of his surgery until this present day (some 15 years later), he virtually has eliminated all obvious sources of fat from his diet and avoids cholesterol-containing foods and unhealthful lifestyle habits. He follows a vigorous, progressive exercise program. For him, insight and the fear of death resulted in his behavioral changes. His new habits have given him a new life—and a stronger character as well.

Strong character and good habits are inseparable.

WHO CAN CHANGE YOUR HABITS?

"No one can persuade another to change," Marilyn Ferguson states in Stephen R. Covey's *The Seven Habits of Highly Effective People*. "Each of us guards a gate of change that can be opened only from the inside. We cannot open the gate of another, either by argument or by emotional appeal."

The *Wall Street Journal* says that Americans today understand more about how to live longer, healthier lives than ever before. People are paying more attention to nutrition labels, eating more low-fat food, and trying to exercise more. Eighty-two percent of the persons who responded to a *Wall Street Journal* health poll said taking care of their health is important to them. And their efforts show: American life expectancy has never been higher; heart disease among the middle-aged has plummeted; and many of the infectious diseases that once killed millions of people have been wiped out.

But the effort has not been easy.

A Johns Hopkins medical letter, *Health After 50*, states, "Only one in five persons who tries to change behavior succeeds the first time. It takes smokers 3-4 attempts before they successfully quit. And weight loss—a change that would benefit more than a third of all Americans—may be the hardest change of all."

Researchers claim that fewer than 20 percent of people with less-than-ideal behavior are prepared to change at any given time.

**If you want more of what you've got,
keep doing what you are doing.
If you want something different,
do something different.**
—Old Proverb

M. Scott Peck writes in his book *In Search of Stones*, "I was foolishly seeking a substitute for God. So it is with virtually all addictions. They are forms of idolatry. For the alcoholic, the bottle becomes an idol; for the heroin addict, the drug is the god. The nondrug addictions are no different. Our whole society may be going down the tubes because of its idolatry of wealth and security."

The first commandment says, "I am the LORD your God. . . . You shall have no other gods before me" (Exod. 20:2-3).

BAD HABITS ARE HARD TO BREAK

Have you ever wondered why bad habits (especially bad lifestyle habits) are so hard to break? It is probably because we become addicted to our lifestyle. Behavioral psychologist John Martin has written extensively on behavioral modification and exercise in the sedentary adult. He states that the sedentary lifestyle with its careless patterns is a true addiction with physiologic and psychologic reactions and thought processes.

The organism (you and I) rejects change because it wants to hold on to what it has. The reality is that we have "worked" for many years to become overweight and underfit. Not only that, but our body chemistry has adapted to that state of being, and our thought patterns compute that way.

Here's the good news: Rats in mazes and chickens in cages change habits—and so can we.

There are five stages of change, according to the Johns Hopkins medical letter *Health After 50*.

1. **Precontemplation** is a potentially long-lasting stage in which the negative aspects of an undesirable behavior (the fact that smoking promotes lung cancer, for example) remain at the periphery of one's mind.

2. **Contemplation** occurs when the person toys with the idea of changing. During this stage the person examines the problem behavior and tries to balance the costs and benefits of changing it. This stage can be lengthy. In one study of 200 smokers, most remained in this stage for two years.

3. **Preparation** unites the intention to change with a plan of action. The individual in this phase intends to take concrete steps to change within the next month and has often unsuccessfully taken action in the previous year.

4. **Action** occurs when actual steps are taken to modify behavior. The action phase can range from one day to six months. The person in this stage feels empowered and in control of his or her life but often relies on support from others.

5. **Maintenance** is the prevention of relapse. It begins six months after taking action and can last a lifetime.

Several cycles through the stages of change are usually required before effective change actually occurs. Change is not impossible, but it is hard.

The key is in developing healthful, wholesome habits.

HELP WITH HABITS—START SIMPLE

None of my five children developed the habit of brushing his or her teeth without help. They are now very good at it. What did we do right?

1. We started *simple*. They had only one or two teeth when we started.

2. We did it *consistently*. We did not decide each day whether it was a good idea or not.

3. We did it by *cues*. It was time to brush teeth when the pajamas were on, right before evening prayers and good-night kisses.

4. We made it *fun*. Motorboat games, different kinds of brushes, a variety of toothpastes, and fancy brush holders, all contributed to the frivolity.

5. *We didn't quit* if we forgot or couldn't brush one night for some reason.

6. We used *positive reinforcement*. I had to cover my eyes when they flashed their postbrushing smiles. Mom was equally proud of their clean, white teeth.

7. We built in long-term *goals* and *rewards*. They would have many years of healthy teeth, pleasant smiles, and no dentist drills.

8. We spent *years in the process*. At five or six years of age they could be trusted to brush their teeth by themselves. I calculate that over the years by brushing their teeth and mine, I have assisted or brushed teeth 47,875 times!

Now, how about your exercise habit?

- Start *simple*—one exercise.
- Do it *consistently*—five days a week.
- Do it by *cues*—a certain time of day, such as when you get up, when you get home, or right before dinner.
- Make it *fun*.
- When you forget or miss, *do not quit.*
- Get *positive reinforcements* by telling yourself you are in control and capable of changing your habits. Your courage, strength, and resolve are admirable to your spouse and/or close friends.
- Your *long-term goal* is to live better with less health problems, increased energy, more confidence, and greater self-esteem. You might live longer as well.

GOOD HABITS AND ACCOUNTABILITY

For one year I exercised faithfully three times a week from 6 to 7 A.M. I earned 4,949 aerobic points, ran 242.5 miles, and cycled 1,840 miles.

That same year for one hour each Saturday morning, I went to my church for a time of prayer and spiritual development. Four early morning meetings a month. How did I do it?

I was *accountable*. A group of four or five people expected me to be there. In fact, they needed me to be there, just as I needed them. Success and adherence to a discipline is greatly increased by accountability. Consider these suggestions:

1. Be accountable to people (or someone) who share(s) your struggle or pursuit. Sign a contract or make a friendly agreement.
2. Set a specific time to meet. Keep it as consistent as possible.
3. Develop individual/group rewards and consequences.
4. Keep a careful log of event, time, and resulting benefits (for example, "walked 2 miles in 40 minutes = 200 calories burned").
5. Tell your friends. Talk tends to motivate you to "put up or shut up."
6. Read articles and materials on your interest (wellness, exercise, spiritual discipline, and so on).
7. Keep personal records. Try to set a new personal record every month or so.
8. Put a map or chart in a visible place in your home or office to record your progress.

Our lives in many ways consist of performing a series of habits good and bad. Lifestyle changes (eliminating bad habits and adopting good ones) is one goal in this book. It takes months to entrench and trust new habits, so don't be discouraged if you lose your good habit for a day or a week. Persevere. Results will come if you stick with it.

Start with simple, easily performed, low-intensity, and short-duration changes. Add complexity, frequency, intensity, and longer duration as time goes on.

Above all, don't be like my friend Susan, who is constantly discouraged. She is overweight and out of shape. She has prayed about her condition, set goals, gone to seminars, read books, and taken pills. Still she has failed over and over again. Her mirror constantly reminds her, "I haven't measured up." "I haven't persevered." "I haven't stood the test." "I haven't been obedient." "I . . . I . . . I . . ."

Do you see how self-centered Susan is? She is constantly focusing on herself. Be it ever so negative, it is still self-focus.

But I have good news for my friend Susan: God is not down on her. In fact, if she never loses a pound or walks a mile, God is still going to love her with an everlasting love. He is still going to live inside her and love other people through her.

MORE HELP WITH GOOD HABITS

Greater than 50 percent of people who turn over a new leaf quit sometime between one and six months. Dieting, stop-smoking programs, exercise regimes, early rising, and going to church, all have high attrition rates.

Adhering to a new, more healthful lifestyle is a step toward wholeness. Fan that small but growing spark, and soon it will become a healthy warm fire.

Talk to your family about paying the price now for a fuller and richer tomorrow by acquiring new, healthful, and good habits. After some heart problems I experienced, I have never had to justify the time I spend on my habit of staying fit. I want to live long enough to support my family, enjoy my kids and grandchildren, and keep my wife from being a long-term widow. The miles I travel today are symbolic of the miles I will travel with my wife and children in the tomorrows. Habits make it happen.

DOCTOR'S ORDERS: RX FOR GOOD HABITS

▶ Set up a new government for *yourself: you* become the dictator of your habits.
▶ Create your *future* by making good decisions *today.*
▶ Persevere—never turn back.
▶ Start with simple changes of which you have control—walking, for example.
▶ Respect and build on your "spiritual moments."
▶ If you fail, start over.
▶ Be consistent.
▶ Make your long-term goals visible.
▶ Develop accountability with someone or a group.
Remember: God loves you from the *inside out.*

Given the numerous health benefits of physical activity, the hazards of being inactive are clear. Physical inactivity is a serious, nationwide problem. Its scope poses a public health challenge for reducing the national burden of unnecessary illness and premature deaths.
—Report of the Surgeon General, 1996

CHAPTER 10

A Word from the Doctor . . .
Fitness

The doctor of the future will give no medicine, but will interest his patients in the care of the human frame, in diet, and in the cause and prevention of disease.
—Thomas Edison

It's still good advice, Thomas!

THE FARM FITNESS CLUB

Thirty-five years ago, what did my family do to stay fit? For one thing, we didn't worry about it, because we didn't know it was important. Exercising for fitness was not a part of our lives. However, we did exercise and were fit.

Our exercise regime included

◆ walking over our entire farm every day to irrigate, fix fences, chase cows, and check crops;

◆ shoveling grain, rocks, and dirt;

- pitching hay, bucking bales, digging ditches, stacking hay, and loading and unloading crops and produce;
- hoeing fields and gardens and spading gardens;
- feeding cows by hand with a pitchfork, feeding and slopping pigs, and feeding chickens;
- milking cows in an old barn where we had to carry milk from each cow to the 10-gallon cans that we then loaded and carried to the road for the milkman;
- mowing lawns with a hand-push reel mower;
- clearing fence lines of weeds with a scythe (not a Weedeater or power mower);
- cleaning barns and chicken houses with forks and shovels.

Those were "the good old days," when exercise and fitness were a way of life. We had callused hands and lean bodies. Today, in the late 20th century, fitness is another duty or task to work into our already busy schedules.

There is an interesting contrast between my son getting ready for his senior year in high school and me at age 17 doing the same thing. How did I get strong and bulk up for football? I purposefully made my work harder. I would see how far I could run to the wagon with a 100-plus-pound bale of hay. I would see how many bales I could get on the wagon in an hour and how far away from the wagon I could throw them. I would run between the bales so I could load them and never have the tractor driver stop.

As I did those tasks, I would motivate myself by thinking about beating the Melba (Idaho) High School football team. Melba crushed us the previous year (my junior year) 56 to 6. I would imagine how hard I would be to tackle if my muscles were as hard as steel. (We beat them 13 to 6.)

Forty-one years later, my 17-year-old son is getting ready for his senior year of sports. He has a fitness trainer who has prescribed a program of serious upper- and lower-extremity weight training exercises for him, which he does at a local fitness club a couple of hours three to five times each week. The club is air conditioned and full of expensive equipment with mirrors on the wall reflecting designer-clad patrons. A far cry from the fields of eastern Oregon.

Where is our society today? Do we have healthy bodies, alert minds, and fulfilled souls as individuals? Observations from my medical practice, and health and fitness literature, as well as experiences of friends, family, and my own tell me that

- we have inadequate energy levels,
- we are out of shape,
- we are often depressed,
- we are too fat,
- we die too young,
- we are anxious,
- we are hostile,
- we have limited dreams,
- we pray tiny prayers,
- we are academically underachieving,
- we are lacking social skills,
- we are emotionally unstable.

If you could take a pill, a treatment, or a cure that would change many of these so-called realities in your life and move you toward wholeness, would you take it? *Would you take the cure?*

Who is responsible for our health? The major portion of responsibility for our destiny lies with us.

- We choose our path.
- We dream our future, but we live it one day at a time.
- We write our autobiography first in our minds, then in our lives hour by hour.
- We are personally responsible for much of our health, our fulfillment, our happiness, our productivity, our wholeness.

Genetics, environment, and outside forces may have responsibility for as much as 20 percent of our health and happiness. The other 80 percent is up to us. I cannot blame my parents, spouse, doctor, church, or vocation for my lack of health, happiness, and wholeness.

WOULD YOU TAKE THE CURE?

- If the cure would help you live better, feel better about yourself, be more relaxed, be less depressed, be less anxious, and be more fulfilled—would you take it?
- If the cure would help you lose weight and keep it off, give you a more streamlined body, give you more energy, and give you better health with fewer days sick—would you take it?

◆ If the cure gave you better sleep, increased lung capacity, increased muscle, greater endurance, better performance, improved digestion function, and increased sexual satisfaction—would you take it?

◆ If the cure gave you a higher level of good cholesterol, a lower level of bad cholesterol, decreased chances of getting cancer, decreased chances of heart attack, decreased chances of strokes, decreased blood pressure, and a slower resting heart rate—would you take it?

THE CURE

The physical cure is endurance (aerobic) exercise—rhythmic, continuous exercise of large muscle groups of the body for at least 20 minutes per day—ideally five to six days per week for 40 minutes and with a slightly hard level of intensity. (See Appendix.)

We desperately need a life of wholeness in which we have an alert mind, a healthy body, and a fulfilled soul. If the movement toward wholeness means taking a frequent dose of "The Cure," I personally will be willing to pound the pavement and log those miles!

The beauty is that I find if I can take charge of one area of my life, control spills over into other areas of my life—body, mind, and soul. My taking the cure and achieving a healthy body is a beginning point in the development of an alert mind and possession of a fulfilled soul. I find that when I am physically active. I pray more, read better books, think bigger thoughts, and dream bigger dreams.

Why don't people take the cure?

◆ *It's hard*—Exercise is often thought of as hard and difficult. "Boy, that was a killer!" they say, or "I thought I'd die!" Isn't it interesting that just maybe this is what will keep us alive?

◆ *It's boring*—"Just how boring is a cemetery?" I wonder. The facts are—you run the first 30 minutes for your body, the second 30 minutes for your soul.

◆ *It takes too much time*—How much time does a heart attack take away from your life and from your activities and from your family? Time spent in exercise and running also comes back in bonus hours of longer life with greater vigor.

◆ *It causes arthritis and injuries*—When done appropriately, running and rhythmic endurance exercises do not increase arthritis or joint complications. In fact, running and endurance exercises protect us from arthritis. They increase muscle control. They induce weight reduction. The nutrition of the cartilage is enhanced by the repetitive squeezing and pumping action of the joint surfaces. *We usually don't wear out—we rust out.*

◆ *Exercise is punishment*—How many times in your own life can you recall when you've heard someone refer to exercise as a disciplinary measure? In physical education class, running laps was punishment.

◆ **The *"I don't, can't, won't" attitude*—**A persistent negative sign.

◆ *I'm embarrassed*—Any casual tour through most fitness facilities allows you to see that we all are somewhere in the process of working toward less fat and more muscles.

◆ *I do not have a place and/or the proper equipment*—A jump rope, a flight of stairs, a vacant lot, a mall, a pad for calisthenics may be your answer.

Who can exercise aerobically?

Virtually anyone who can walk a mile can run a marathon. But you must start low and go slow. Whether you are 10, 50, or 80 years old, you can increase your activities. The critical years are the 20- to 40-year age group. During this time you are developing life habits, and it is during this time in life when cardiovascular heart disease can develop and is significantly higher in less active people. The "who" really becomes anyone who is willing to make an inner commitment.

Why should I take the cure?

◆ *Why die when you can live?* Each hour spent in exercise on the average increases one's longevity by two to four hours. That is an outstanding return on your investment. When you begin to exercise and do it faithfully, you have many days and weeks of extra life to enjoy and make your unique contribution.

One study published in the April 19, 1995, issue of the *Journal of the American Medical Association* involved nearly 10,000 men and documented that the highest death rate was among men who were the least fit. The lowest death rate was among men who were the most physically fit. During this study, those who increased their fitness level were able to reduce their mortality risk.

◆ *Why have a diseased heart when you can have a healthy one?* There were 340 people in the control group and 340 people in the study group of a Johns Hopkins University study that documented that activity decreases the risk of heart disease. Described by Gerald T. O'Connor in the 1995 issue of the *American Journal of Epidemiology,* it proved that men in the most active category who were involved in moderate to vigorous exercise had the least risk of coronary artery disease, while those who were the least active had the highest risk of coronary artery disease. This study additionally indicated that the good cholesterol (HDL) level is much more apt to improve with vigorous exercise activity than with less vigorous activities.

◆ *Why not avoid cancer?* Endurance exercises reduce the risk of colon cancer, according to research in the September 21, 1994, issue of the *Journal of the National Cancer Institute.* Another study of 545 women from the Centers for Disease Control confirmed that exercise was a factor in preventing breast, endometrial, and ovarian cancer. These are estrogen-dependent cancers and are among the leading causes of mortality in American women. Physically active women in America, Switzerland, Italy, Finland, and China had a decreased chance of estrogen-dependent cancers compared to their sedentary counterparts. This study further documents that physical activity enhances the natural immune function and seems to stimulate other healthful lifestyle habits.

◆ *Why have a stroke?* A study of 73,000 women nurses, published in the September 1995 *Wellness Health Letter,* indicated that those who were the most physically active had a 42 percent lower risk of stroke and a 44 percent lower risk of heart attack than those who were sedentary. This study suggests that for women, light exercise is better than being sedentary, moderate exercise is better than light exercise, and vigorous exercise is best of all.

◆ *Why experience anxiety and depression?* Regular physical activity improves mood, helps relieve depression, and increases feelings of well-being. This was reported in the Surgeon General's Report on Physical Activity and Health, recorded in the *Physical Activity and Fitness Research Digest* of July 1996.

◆ *Why be flabby?* The 100-calorie-a-day miracle is a miracle. If we burn an extra 100 calories a day with physical activity and still eat the same number of calories, in a month's time we will lose a pound of weight. The fact is, however, that after age 20 the average American puts on two pounds of fat per year for 20 to 30 years or more.

◆ *Why not be more productive and have less absenteeism from work?* People who are physically fit and active take fewer sick-leave days and are less likely to die during their work career.

◆ *Why not get well instead of staying sick?* Studies confirm that exercise enhances the body's natural defenses (killer cells) in young and old persons and in people with AIDS. Natural killer cell activity appears to be very important in the prevention of infections and tumors, according to the 1991 edition of the *International Journal of Sports Medicine.*

Another study on lifestyle changes, reported by Dean Ornish in the May 15, 1991, issue of *Hospital Practice,* indicates that an intensive modification of diet, plus stress management, smoking cessation, and moderate exercise can stop and even reverse the progression of coronary arteriosclerosis.

◆ *Why not believe the Surgeon General's Report on Physical Activity and Health?*

The surgeon general's report states that regular physical activity that is performed on most days of the week reduces the risk of developing or dying from the leading causes of illness and death in the United States.

In addition, exercise

—reduces the risk of developing diabetes;

—reduces the risk of developing high blood pressure;

—helps reduce blood pressure in people who already have high blood pressure;

—helps build and maintain healthy bones, muscles, and joints;

—helps older adults become stronger and better able to move about without falling.

People who are usually inactive can improve their health and well-being by becoming even moderately active on a regular basis. The physical activity need not be strenuous to achieve health benefits, but greater health benefits can be achieved by increasing the amount (duration, frequency, or intensity) of physical activity.

CONCLUSIONS

You can do nothing about your chronological age, but you can do wonders about your physiological age. "You cannot turn the clock back, but you can wind it up again. . . . Exercise is the key with which you wind it," according to Thomas Cureton of the University of Illinois.

Good health and fitness are only a part of life—not the focus of our existence. A balanced life of wholeness includes a healthy body, an alert mind, and a fulfilled soul. Exercise is important in achieving this.

First Tim. 4:7-8 says, "Train yourself to be godly. For physical training is of some value, but godliness has value for all things, holding promise for both the present life and the life to come."

The apostle Paul said, "Do you not know your body is a temple of the Holy Spirit? . . . you were bought at a price; Therefore honor God with your body" (1 Cor. 6:19-20).

DOCTOR'S ORDERS: RX FOR PHYSICAL FITNESS

▶ Get off the sofa.

▶ Put on your shoes.

▶ Head for the street or gym.

▶ Start cautiously, two to three days per week.

▶ Progress slowly until you have reached five to six days per week.

Many of life's failures are persons who did not realize
how close they were to success when they gave up.

C H A P T E R   11

A WORD FROM THE DOCTOR . . .

EXERCISE

I was the health and fitness guru, and they were my fluffy, 40-ish, fatigued disciples. I was a zealous fitness believer armed with personal fitness success, scientific facts, much energy, and a strong desire to help my friends succeed and attain what they were dreaming and truly destined for: success, health, fitness, and longevity.

From a physical standpoint, the "gang of five" was a pretty sorry bunch. Most of them had significant paunches. They all had high cholesterol and high triglycerides. They were considerably overweight, and several had hypertension. None of them were fit, and their exercise regimens ranged from none to sporadic—with an occasional softball game, a rare round of golf, a hunting trip once or twice a year, and basketball or volleyball at a company or church picnic. They were in high-stress positions on the corporate ladder or self-employed with a full burden of responsibilities.

We did fitness testing in which we measured resting pulse rates, blood pressure, percent body fat, flexibility, and strength testing, and we included a modified treadmill stress test. We tested their blood for good and bad cholesterol. We had informational and motivational meetings, distributed log books to record activities, and established accountability.

As you might guess, the "gang of five" experienced substantial success for weeks and months. Three mornings a week they met me (the charged-up cheerleader) at 6 A.M. in the workout facility. It was a great experience:

- ◆ Camaraderie
- ◆ Exercises
- ◆ Accountability
- ◆ Encouragement
- ◆ Shared experiences

We all attended the same church, so the spiritual aspects of being fit and vital to serve a needy community with the Good News also motivated us.

The "gang" lost weight, dropped their cholesterol levels, bought smaller belts, felt younger, and had a new sense of self-esteem and confidence.

In time, I sold the physical-therapy practice with the workout facility. Family, job, and time commitments slowly eroded into our mornings, and the "gang of five" disbanded. We all went our own, less-healthy ways. I am sad to report that none of us are quite at the same fitness level we were then.

Exercise is essential for fitness and health. The "gang of five" proved that, and some of the "backsliders" are proving that fitness is lost without exercise.

Success is 10 percent inspiration and 90 percent perspiration.

WHAT IS PHYSICAL FITNESS?

Fitness fact: physical fitness is not a static state of being. It is a process.

Physical fitness, according to a 1971 report from the President's Council on Physical Fitness and Sports, is "the ability to carry out daily tasks with vigor and alertness, without undue fatigue and with ample energy to enjoy leisure-time pursuits and to meet unforeseen emergencies." Physical fitness is not a static state of being that can be stored up. It is a process, a dynamic way of life.

The identifiable components of physical fitness that can be measured, defined, and developed are listed by David C. Nieman in *The Sports Medicine Fitness Course*. They are as follows:

1. *Cardiorespiratory, aerobic fitness:* a strong heart and lungs, a healthy circulatory tree, and muscles with a well-developed system to take in and utilize oxygen for energy purposes.

2. *Body composition:* an appropriate amount of fat and lean body tissue. Obesity is an excessive accumulation of fat.

3. *Musculoskeletal endurance:* the ability for trained muscles to sustain submaximal force repeatedly or for long times. For example, the number of push-ups you can do in one minute.

4. *Musculoskeletal flexibility:* the ability or capacity of the joints to move through a full range of motion.

5. *Musculoskeletal strength:* the maximum force that can be exerted against resistance. For example, the maximum weight one can lift in a bench press.

6. *Other components of physical fitness:* agility, balance, coordination, speed, and reaction time. Even though skill-related fitness is important for athletic performance, it has less to do with general health and longevity. You can be healthy and not athletic, and you can be athletic but not healthy.

Success is not a destination . . . it is a road (so keep on moving).

THE IMPORTANCE OF AEROBIC FITNESS

Aerobic means "in the presence of oxygen," as contrasted with *anaerobic,* which means "in the absence of oxygen."

Aerobic has to do with the utilization of oxygen. Aerobic exercises are activities performed with sufficient duration, intensity, and frequency to effect beneficial changes in the heart, lungs, and vascular system. As we become aerobically fit, our lungs develop a greater capacity, and our blood becomes more efficient in absorbing and transporting oxygen. Muscles, including the heart muscles, become larger and capable of greater endurance. This allows maximum body performance with the least amount of energy expended, resulting in less fatigue and greater productivity.

Just as fire burns with more vigor when fanned (which forces oxygen into the flame), so do our muscles work better in the presence of oxygen—in fact, 13 times better.

That is why when you become aerobically fit you have so much more energy at the end of the day.

Success is more attitude than aptitude.

PHYSICAL ACTIVITY INDEX*

Fitness fact: the best exercises are the ones you do.

Just how active are you? Take the following test. A high score means a potential for a lot of good living.

****

PHYSICAL ACTIVITY INDEX

Calculate your activity index by multiplying your score for each category (Score = intensity x duration x frequency):

	Score	*Activity*
Intensity	5	Sustained heavy breathing and perspiration
	4	Intermittent heavy breathing and perspiration—as in tennis or racquetball
	3	Moderately heavy—as in recreational sports and cycling
	2	Moderate—as in volleyball, softball
	1	Light—as in fishing, walking
Duration	4	Over 30 minutes
	3	20-30 minutes
	2	10-20 minutes
	1	Under 10 minutes
Frequency	5	Daily or almost daily
	4	3-5 times a week
	3	1-2 times a week
	2	Few times a month
	1	Less than once a month

Score	*Evaluation*	*Fitness Category*
100	Very active lifestyle	High
60-80	Active and healthy	Very good
40-60	Acceptable (could be better)	Fair
20-40	Not good enough	Poor
Under 20	Sedentary	Very poor

If you scored in the "very poor," "poor," or "fair" range, do not despair. Start low, go slow. Persevere, and you can succeed.

*Brian J. Sharkey, Ph.D., *Physiology of Fitness,* 2nd ed. (Champaign, Ill.: Human Kinetics Publishers, 1984).

Body Wisdom

Fitness fact: the body seems to have the wisdom to send
appropriate messages about work and play.

I am a firm believer in "body wisdom." At an appropriate time in the treatment of my patients, I often ask, "Are you ready to return to work, sports, or some other activity?" The amazing thing is that the answer is usually prompt and decisive. The body seems to have the "wisdom" to send appropriate messages about work and play.

In regard to exercise, if your body wisdom says yes, you could probably start today. However, it may be in your best interest to complete the questionnaire in Appendix 1.

**It is easier to go down a hill than up,
but the view is better from the top.**

Start Low—Go Slow

Fitness fact: the "start low—go slow" principle
applies to almost every area of life, especially physical fitness.

The other night a friend who is a banker made an astonishing statement: "If you gave your child one penny for his first birthday and doubled each previous year's amount on every birthday afterwards, by age 28 he would be receiving over a million dollars on each birthday." I challenged him to prove it. He did.

Our son L. D.'s first ascent of 14,000-plus-foot-high Mount Rainier in Washington state was accomplished in one day. But not really. Every day for many weeks he had made multiple, little, difficult steps up a 100-yard steep hill with boots and a heavy pack on his back. He started *low* and went *slow*, increasing his efforts daily. One day he climbed out of bed at 2 A.M. at Camp Muir and got dressed for the picture at the top of Mount Rainier. Those daily ascents of the 100-yard hill were a real part of the final climb to the summit.

The "start low—go slow" principle applies to almost every area of life, including physical fitness. If you start with a one-eighth-mile walk and double the distance every two months, in one year you will be walking eight miles per workout. But in exercise, rather than doubling your efforts, a more prudent approach would be to add to your efforts. For instance, starting with a quarter-mile walk or jog and increasing the distance by a quarter mile every month would have you walking or jogging three miles each workout by the end of a year.

Certainly there are limits out there for all of us—but we do not know where they are until we get closer to them. If we start low and go slow, we will find that some of our limits were only imagined.

The "start low—go slow" principle is especially important to you and your physical fitness if you have a medical history of high cholesterol, hypertension, diabetes, obesity, or heart disease; if you have family members who have had heart attacks at an early age; if you smoke; or if you are over 40 years old with an inactive lifestyle.

We may have laughed at the tortoise in the fable, "The Tortoise and the Hare"—until we read the last paragraph. The "start low—go slow" tortoise who stuck with it was and still is the winner.

Success is a marathon, not a sprint.

ACTIVITY GOALS

Fitness fact: Do not set weight loss goals; set activity goals.

After many years of faithful aerobic exercise, I enjoy excellent aerobic conditioning. At the present time I do not feel I need or want to increase my conditioning program.

However, if you are just beginning your aerobic journey and need more direction on how to keep your body improving, the American Orthopaedic Society for Sports Medicine has devised an acronym for fitness: FITTS.

F = frequency of aerobic training.

I = intensity of aerobic training.

T = amount of time spent training.

T = type of exercises.

S = speed or the rate of progression of aerobic exercise.

THE *F* OF FITTS

Fitness fact: fitness is improved by exercising four or five days a week.
F stands for **frequency,** or the number of times per week.

Any exercise is better than no exercise. However, for cardiovascular and muscular conditioning, three nonconsecutive days are considered the absolute minimum frequency per week to maintain aerobic conditioning. Fitness improves rapidly with each day up to three days a week. There is additional improvement with additional days but at a slower rate. It would be best to consider four to five days a week as a minimum requirement. In that way, if you miss a day or two, the three-day minimum is still met.

Frequency can be increased for a specific purpose, such as accelerating a weight loss program. Effective weight loss may require six to seven workouts a week with longer durations. But the increased chances of injury must be taken seriously.

One way frequency can be increased safely is by using alternate cross-training techniques: biking one day, running on the opposite day, and so on. Additionally, you can safely increase intensity with the easy-hard principle, such as walking three miles one day and jogging five miles the next.

Frequency can be one of the most difficult hurdles you will experience in becoming fit. As with any task, the beginning requires a tough mind-set. Getting dressed and started is 90 percent of the battle. After that, the "enchantment" of the dance will carry you along.

**Faith does not demand that we win;
it does demand that we keep trying.**

THE *I* OF FITTS

*Fitness fact: the intensity of your aerobic exercise
should be enough to maintain the heart rate between 60 percent
and 85 percent of your predicted maximum heart rate.*
I stands for **intensity** of aerobic training.

Aerobic exercise should maintain the heart rate at between 60 percent and 85 percent of the predicted maximum heart rate. Below that level, little training effect occurs, and anything above that level represents an increased danger for both injury and potential cardiovascular problems.

There are several ways to determine your exercise intensity. The *perceived exertion scale* is one of them. On the perceived exertion scale you should be in the very light to somewhat hard range. This will give you a pulse rate of approximately 90 to 150.

The *talk test* is another way to test your level of intensity. You should exercise to the point just below where you start to get breathless when talking. If you can't talk, slow down.

Enjoyment is often directly related to intensity. If you are attempting to go too fast too soon or too slow too long, you will not get maximum enjoyment (or maximum benefit) from exercising. It has been my impression during the course of a run, whether 2 or 10 miles, I get the greatest enjoyment when I am well into my training heart range.

If you are going to err on intensity, err on the low side and perform your activity longer.

THE FIRST *T* OF FITTS

Fitness fact: if you are in a hurry to get in shape, exercise longer, not harder.
T stands for **time** spent training.

Your weekly *minimum* duration goal should be at least one and a half to two hours of cardiovascular training. This is actual aerobic training time (keeping the heart rate between 60 percent and 85 percent of the predicted maximum heart rate) and does not include warming up, stretching, or cooling down. The target (or training) heart rate is based upon one's predicted maximum heart rate. The most accurate and expensive method to determine the predicted maximum heart rate is to perform a maximum-stress treadmill test. However, if you are unable to do the treadmill test, I suggest using formulas and/or charts to determine your predicted maximum heart rate and your target heart rate. See page 270 of *The Aerobic Program for Total Well-Being* by Kenneth Cooper.

Early in your training program you will not be able to do as much as you would like, but with improved conditioning it will be possible. A training session should include three periods:

1. *The warm-up period.* A warm-up is light walking or jogging, easy calisthenics, or stretching exercises. These prepare the body, the muscles, ligaments, and heart for the more vigorous activity to come. Regardless of your age or level of fitness, failure to warm up before exercise can result in electrocardiogram abnormalities, notes Brian J. Sharkey in *Physiology of Fitness.* A simple four- or five-minute slow jog is a great warm-up and will generally prevent any such problems, he says.

2. *The aerobic period.* During the aerobic period the heart rate should be kept within the target zone. Remember: there is an inverse relationship between exercise intensity and duration. In other words, the lighter the activity, the longer it must be maintained to be aerobically beneficial. The more intense the activity, the less time it requires

for aerobic benefit. An activity that is light enough to be performed for at least 30 to 40 minutes is recommended. Activity more intense (and thus shorter) than that results in less improvement and potential increased risk of injury.

3. **The cooldown period.** Don't stop all at once! Bring the body back from exercise slowly. If you simply stop, light-headedness and passing out can occur. Also, never go directly from a workout to a hot shower, sauna, or hot tub. Your core temperature may be 100 to 104 degrees from exercise, and increased heat may be unsafe.

If you must lie down after exercise, put your feet up. As much as 70 percent of your circulating blood may be below your waist following a vigorous jog.

Remember: even Olympic champions take a slow victory lap following the competition. This does more than simply please the crowd; it is a prudent way to cool down.

After your aerobic workout today, take a victory lap. Wave to the adoring, cheering crowd. Do some stretching, relax a few minutes, drink a glass of cool water. Then hit the shower and congratulate yourself.

The best time to do something is between yesterday and tomorrow.

THE SECOND *T* OF FITTS

Fitness fact: the best exercise is the one you will do.
T stands for **type** of exercise.

Everyone is looking for the perfect exercise. I suggest you choose an activity or a group of activities you enjoy. The best exercise is the one that keeps you coming back for more. Recent scientific tests seem to indicate that after all is said and done, the treadmill is probably the basic Cadillac for fitness training. It is safe, everyone seems to know how to use it, it demands that you keep up with a certain preset pace, and when you walk briskly and swing your arms vigorously, it is an excellent workout.

Besides the treadmill, other good aerobic exercises are cross-country running, cycling, swimming, stairsteppers, aerobic dance, and in-line skating. The point is you need to exercise at a level of activity that will burn 7.5 calories per minute or more or be on your perceived exertional level at the point at which you are receiving maximum benefit.

THE *S* OF FITTS

Fitness fact: if your rate of progression is slow and sensible,
your new level of activity will enhance, not threaten, your health.

S stands for **speed** or the rate of progression of aerobic exercise.

Most people start out too fast. How many times have you started a program of jogging, cycling, or swimming and been unable to get out of bed the next morning? Not only starting out too fast but progressing too rapidly increases the risk of an overuse injury. Little-by-little progression may seem too slow, but it allows for surprisingly rapid improvement in aerobic fitness while minimizing stress on the body.

The best advice for those who wish to improve their fitness level is to increase only one of the three training variables (FIT—frequency, intensity, time) at a time. For example, don't go directly from three 30-minute workouts to four 40-minute workouts. See Appendix 2.

> **The sum of the whole is this: walk and be happy, walk and be healthy. The best way to lengthen out our days is to walk steadily and with purpose.**
> —Charles Dickens

THE RESTING HEART RATE IS IMPORTANT

Fitness fact: a slow heart rate is important,
because the heart rests only between beats.

In a year's time the fit heart (at 60 beats per minute) beats 10,512,000 fewer times than the unfit heart (at 80 beats per minute). Consider the millions of extra times the unfit heart must beat in a lifetime.

It is obvious that the body is not always at rest, but the resting heart rate is an indicator of the heart rate in general. That is, a person with a low resting heart rate also has a lower heart rate while working and playing.

Besides by regular aerobic exercise, the heart rate can be lowered by reducing body fat (less tissue to pump blood to and through) and by decreasing stress.

Although some highly conditioned endurance athletes have resting heart rates as low as 30 to 40 beats per minute, 60 beats per minute is a reasonable and attainable goal for the average person.

IS EXERCISE SAFE?

Fitness fact: progressive, regular, moderate exercise is safe and protective.

Yes—exercise is safe. The small risk can be nearly eliminated if you remember the following:

1. Stay below fatigue level. "Perceived exertion" (how you feel) may be as important as your target heart rate.
2. Stop before exhaustion.
3. Start your exercise program at low intensity, and progress slowly.
4. Be consistent, three to five times per week.
5. Long, slow distances and moderate exercises are better than short, fast, high-intensity activities.
6. If you work out infrequently, or if it has been more than three weeks, begin again and proceed slowly.
7. If you are an infrequent, intense type A exerciser with multiple risk factors (overweight, smoker, high blood pressure, high cholesterol), you are an accident waiting to happen. Get medical clearance.

CALORIES: I CAN RELATE TO THAT!

Fitness fact: the key to weight control is exercise.

An overweight and out-of-shape friend of mine faithfully, dutifully, and reluctantly met me three times each week to earn aerobic points. As the weeks went by, he trimmed up, began to use the fitness lingo, and improved his aerobic conditioning remarkably. But when it was time to work out on his own without my prodding and direction, he faltered.

Looking back, I wonder if he would have persisted if he had related his workouts to calorie burn-up rather than aerobic points. I don't think cardiovascular fitness, important as it is, was nearly as significant to him as controlling his weight. Since he had always seen himself as "the fat little boy," an emphasis on calorie consumption may have made him more intense and persistent.

Regular workouts that burn more than 300 calories decrease serum cholesterol and triglyceride levels, assisting in weight control and fat metabolism.

According to the theory of aerodynamics as may
be readily demonstrated through wind tunnel
experiments, the bumblebee is unable to fly.
This is because the weight, size, and shape of its
body in relation to the total wingspread makes
flying impossible. But the bumblebee, being
ignorant of these scientific truths, goes ahead and
flies anyway and makes a little honey every day.
—Anonymous

◆ The goal of a calorie-based exercise program is to burn at least 2,000 calories a week in planned aerobic exercise. This should be spread out over three to five days. If only three days, they should be nonconsecutive.
◆ The best results are achieved if you burn at least 7.5 calories per minute. (Walking a mile in 13 to 14 minutes would achieve this.)
◆ Unfit individuals should start with workouts of 100 to 200 calories.
◆ Fit individuals can have workouts of 200 to 400 calories.
◆ Very fit individuals can have workouts of 400-plus calories.

See Appendix 3 for a chart giving you an idea of how many calories are burned performing various activities, and Appendix 4 for an interesting "Exercise Across America" challenge.

THE GOOD NEWS ABOUT STRENGTH TRAINING

(Adapted from the Johns Hopkins Medical Letter: Health After 50, April 1997)

First some bad news: By age 70, most people have 20 to 30 percent less muscle tissue than they did at age 30. This slow process of erosion has recently been recognized as a bonafide medical condition called sacropenia, which means "vanishing flesh."

Sacropenia has significant health implications because it impairs balance and limits strength. Together, these two developments increase the likelihood of falls, which produce bone fractures. Broken bones are a leading cause of disability and death. Osteoporosis (weak bones that break easily) develops at about the same pace as sacropenia. Osteoporosis occurs in all of us but is greatly exaggerated in the inactive person.

Now the good news: Both endurance and strength training are helpful in the prevention of osteoporosis.

The effects of weak muscles can be significantly reduced and even reversed by moderate amounts of strength training (also called resistance training, power training, or weight training) targeting specific muscles.

Strength training is any type of exercise performed in order to increase the strength and bulk of specific muscles. Strength training is usually performed in one place while standing, sitting, or lying down. Exercises can be performed by using free weights or weight machines or by working against gravity. Leg lifts, arm curls, and abdominal crunches are a few examples of strength-training exercises.

The goal of strength training is to challenge the targeted muscles by performing at least three sets of 8 to 12 repetitions and to gradually increase the amount of weight used.

Strength training significantly slows the inevitable loss of muscle mass (sacropenia) with aging (½ percent vs. 1 percent per year).

Other benefits of strength training are

increased metabolism,

increased bone density,

decreased risk of diabetes,

better ratio of "good" (HDL) cholesterol to "bad" (LDL) cholesterol,

pain relief for osteoarthritis and possible rheumatoid arthritis.

CONCLUSION

After 33 years of medical practice, I have learned some valuable lessons about wholeness. That is why I keep pounding the "aerobic fitness drum." Our physical well-being is far more important to us than we are generally willing to admit.

◆ Fitness is a factor in our wholeness equation that we can control—it is present tense and modifiable.

◆ Our fitness level has a tremendous positive or negative impact on all the other areas of our lives.

◆ Poor health is devastating to a productive, full life.

◆ Premature and/or preventable death is a profound and far-reaching loss.

My father-in-law died from heart disease after a long and difficult postsurgery course. It could not have been much worse: severe chest pain, an emergency visit to the hospital, emergency angioplasty to try to open occluded previous bypass surgery heart vessels, failed angioplasty, emergency open-heart surgery while on blood thinners, severe blood loss with the long, complex surgery, touch and go waiting for days while he was in a coma, deterioration, multiple systems failure—and finally, after 30 days, death.

I am certain that this godly man could have easily lived several additional years. I wish that he had known about fitness, wellness, aerobic exercise, healthful diet, and healthful lifestyle in his adult years. His death was a great loss to me, our family, our friends, our church, and our community.

My plea is for good, decent, hardworking, salt-of-the-earth, godly people to become fully alive. We need healthy, fulfilled, holy people on every street, in every city, living long, productive lives of wholeness.

Doctor's Orders: Rx for Exercise

▶ Exercise four to five times per week for 40 to 60 minutes.

▶ Focus on endurance exercises, but do not exclude strength training.

▶ Save lots of money for your long, active, productive, enjoyable retirement years.

We could postpone 75% of deaths through lifestyle changes, compared to just 15% by advanced medical procedures.

—C. Everett Koop
former United States surgeon general

CHAPTER 12

A WORD FROM THE DOCTOR . . .

WEIGHT CONTROL

Jerry and I were born five minutes apart on April 6, 1938. I was the firstborn and weighed five pounds. Jerry weighed four pounds. Through our growing-up years we lived together, worked together, played together, and ate together. We married and went our separate ways. We have stayed in shape, tried to deal with stress in our lives, have great marriages, and enjoy fulfilling lives. We enjoy emotional, physical, and mental health.

Will we die at, or very near, the same age? Will I precede my brother in death by five minutes? Since I weigh 173 pounds and Jerry weighs 160, his cholesterol should be about 12 points better than mine, which means his chance of premature death from cardiovascular disease is less. He probably has 2 to 3 points lower blood pressure and has a slightly lower chance of having cancer because he eats less fat and makes better food choices.

FATTENING OF AMERICA: CURRENT STATE OF AFFAIRS

Obesity refers specifically to having excess body fat. Experts generally agree that men with more than 25 percent body fat and women with more than 30 percent body fat are obese.

◆ Greater than 30 percent of Americans are obese.

◆ 71 percent of Americans over 25 years of age are obese.

◆ The economic cost of obesity in America is well over $100 billion per year. Over half of those costs are direct medical costs, while the rest are related to lost workdays and the purchasing of diet and weight loss programs and products.

Obesity is not a cosmetic problem; it is a health problem.

◆ Obesity is related to 5 of the 10 leading causes of death:

◆ Heart disease

◆ Stroke

◆ Hypertension

◆ Diabetes

◆ Cancer (In men this includes cancer of the colon, rectum, and prostate; and in women, cancer of the gallbladder, breast, uterus, cervix, and ovaries.)

◆ In addition, obesity causes an increased risk of early death,
gallbladder disease,
increased gout,
orthopedic problems with arthritis,
orthopedic problems with back disease,
abdominal hernia,
complications in surgery secondary to tissue healing,
surgical complications,
postoperative infections,
problems with pregnancy,
falls due to loss of agility and mobility,
problems with sleep apnea,
pulmonary problems,
psychological burdens.

WHAT CAUSES OBESITY?

All living organisms are driven by a constant demand for energy. Plants trap energy from sunlight, while all other life forms stay alive by oxidizing (metabolizing) foodstuffs.

Our body converts the food we eat into sugars, amino acids (proteins), and fats that are transported by our blood to cells.

Nature is generous. When you begin to sit around, she provides more cushions.
—Anonymous

Everyone needs a certain amount of body fat for stored energy, heat and insulation, shock absorption, and other functions. As a rule, women have more fat than men. Obesity occurs when a person's calorie intake exceeds the amount of energy he or she burns. Evidence suggests that obesity often has more than one cause. Genetic, environmental, psychological, and other factors, all play a part.

Genetic **factors in obesity:** Obesity tends to run in families, suggesting a genetic cause. The so-called obesity gene is getting a lot of publicity in the press and on television, fueling the scorn of those who believe that the call for proper eating and more physical activity is a waste of time, because "if you're destined to be fat and unfit, so be it." But the evidence says that the leading causes of premature death (and a lot of unhealthy misery during life) are smoking, obesity, and inactivity. *These are personal choices.*

Research confirms that there is a significant genetic factor involved in being overweight *for some people.* However, in more than 50 percent of overweight people, genetics is not the main reason—lifestyle habits are the reason.

Environmental **factors in obesity:** Lifestyle behaviors, such as what people eat and how active they are, determine how likely it is they will lose weight. Some people have been able to lose weight and keep it off by

- ◆ learning how to choose more nutritious meals that are lower in fat;
- ◆ learning to recognize environmental cues (such as enticing smells) that may make them want to eat when they are not hungry;
- ◆ becoming more physically active.

Psychological **factors in obesity:** Many people eat in response to negative emotions such as boredom, sadness, or anger.

While most overweight people do not have more psychological problems than normal weight people, about 30 percent of the people who seek treatment for serious weight problems have difficulties with binge eating.

The pain of remaining the same is greater than the pain of change.

In this century, outward appearance has become more important than inner character, because sexual attractiveness has replaced spirituality as the most important attribute of a woman, according to John P. Forest and G. Ken Goodrick in *Living Without Dieting*. Many people accept society's standards of attractiveness and body size. When they fail to meet these standards, they are troubled.

Other causes of obesity: Other causes of obesity include some very rare illnesses, such as hypothyroidism, Cushing's syndrome, depression, and certain neurological problems that lead to overeating. It should be noted, however, that fewer than 1 percent of all causes of obesity are on the basis of a true medical abnormality. Some drugs, including steroids and some antidepressants, may also cause weight gain.

How Do We Measure Body Fat?

Precisely measuring the body's fat is not easy, but some of the methods used are as follows:

1. *Underwater weighing.* This sophisticated technique is the gold standard, but a special laboratory is needed, and it can be expensive.
2. *Skin fold or skin caliper measurements.* This technique is quite accurate, readily available, and usually inexpensive.
3. *Bioelectric impedance analysis.* This is not as available, requires a bit more expense, and is not as reliable as other means.
4. *Weight-for-height tables.* See Appendix 5.
5. *Body mass index.* Body mass index uses a mathematical formula that takes into account both a person's height and weight. See Appendix 6.
6. *Weight formulas.* According to the October 1996 edition of *Sports Medicine*, the weight-measuring formula for women is

100 pounds for the first 5 feet in height plus 4 to 5 pounds for every inch thereafter; for men the formula is 106 pounds for the first 5 feet plus 5 to 6 pounds for every inch thereafter. This formula, however, does not account for bone structure and musculature, so add or subtract 10 percent or so if you have a large or small bone or muscle structure.

It is better to be a "pear" than an "apple."

7. *Waist-to-hip ratio.* As doctors, we are concerned with not only how much fat a person has, but also where that fat is located. Women typically collect fat in their hips and buttocks, giving their figures a "pear" shape. Men, on the other hand, usually build up fat around their bellies, giving them more of an "apple" shape. Obviously, this is not a hard-and-fast rule. Some men are pear shaped, and some women become apple shaped, especially after menopause.

   People whose fat is concentrated mostly in the abdomen are more likely to develop many of the health problems associated with obesity.

   Doctors have developed a simple way to measure whether someone is an apple or a pear. The measurement is called the waist-to-hip ratio.

   To calculate someone's waist-to-hip ratio, measure the waist, then measure the hips at the widest point. Divide the waist measurement by the hip measurement. A woman with a 35-inch waist and 46-inch hips would do the following calculation: 35 divided by 46 = 0.76. Women with waist-to-hip ratios of more than 0.8 or men with waist-to-hip ratios of more than 1.0 are "apples." They are at increased health risk because of their fat distribution.

8. *Pinch an inch!* If you can pinch greater than an inch midway between your belly button and your side at waist level while standing, you may need to lose weight.

HOW IS OBESITY TREATED?

1. *DIET:* Your diet should contain about 60 percent complex carbohydrates, 25 to 30 percent fats, another 15 percent proteins. You should not have an excessively low-calorie diet, and you need a variety of foods. It is probably wise to supplement your diet with a good multivitamin. Ideally you will eat more of your food in the early part of the day rather than later. Your diet cannot in and of itself be effective for long-term weight reduction. For true success you must add exercise.

GARDEN OF EDEN DIET

A "perfect world" diet: In an imperfect world, what is a perfect diet? The simple answer is that we don't really know, but it would no doubt look like, smell like, and feel like the gourmet food served in the Garden of Eden, the perfect world (see Gen. 1:29). Fresh vegetables, grains, nuts, and fruits were the daily fare. It was only after the flood in Gen. 9:3 that people became omnivorous (plant-plus-animal food sources).

Our present knowledge and understanding of nutrition suggest that a healthful diet consists of lots of grains, vegetables, and fruits, with the option of lesser amounts of meat and / or animal product foods.

Fluids should include plenty of pure water, as well as nutritional drinks such as juices and nonfat milks. Coffee and tea are permissible in small amounts.

It is my opinion that alcohol in any form is not justified, given the societal and physiological problems surrounding it. Just one ounce of alcohol will suppress cell functions in the body, including brain and nerve cells. There is no medicinal or protective worth from alcohol that adequately offsets these poisoning effects on our brain and nerve cells.

How many calories do we need? We all need enough calories to sustain a vigorous lifestyle and maintain an appropriate weight.

How do I calculate the number of calories I need? If you multiply your weight by 15, that is approximately the number of calories you need to maintain your weight. So, if you weigh 200 pounds, you will need 3,000 calories (200 x 15) to maintain your current weight, assuming you have a normal activity program. If you need to gain weight, you would eat a few more calories. If you are unusually active with workouts and hard work, you should take in additional calories to maintain your weight. If you want to lose weight, then you would eat fewer calories than are needed to maintain your weight.

If I want to lose weight, how much should I eat? Let's assume that you weigh 200 pounds and want to get down to 180 pounds. What should your calorie consumption be? Remember the formula: desired weight x 15 = calories needed to maintain that weight. So 180 x 15 = 2,700 calories. Again, it is safe to assume that you have been consuming 3,000 calories a day to maintain your 200-pound weight, so your weight loss diet will contain 300 calories fewer. Since 1 pound of fat contains 3,500 calories, it will take you 12 to 15 days to lose 1 pound of fat. That's approximately 2 pounds a month. With the addition of the slightest amount of exercise above and beyond your current activity level, you could lose even more.

How much fat should be in my diet? Thirty percent *or less* of your calorie intake should be in the form of fat. (30 percent is a high estimate, particularly if there is any history of cancer or cholesterol problems. Some specialists believe that it might be best to be as low as 10-15 percent.) If you divide your weight by two, that is about the number of grams of fat you could eat each day. So if you weigh 200 pounds, you can eat 100 grams of fat (200 ÷ 2 = 100). Since there are 9 calories in every gram of fat, that gives you 900 calories of fat in your 3,000-calorie-a-day diet.

How about highly processed foods? If foods are highly processed, they are also usually high in fat, sodium, preservatives, and/or simple sugars. Avoid these foods. If you simply *must* eat them, get back to the garden as quickly as you can.

How much and how fast should I lose weight? Never attempt to lose more than 10 percent of your weight at any one time. After you achieve that goal, then reset and recalculate your commitment to weight reduction.

2. DRUGS: New drugs for weight reduction are available. Exactly how safe they are and how many complications are going to result over the long haul is yet to be determined. Drugs should be something you take only after seeing your physician and consulting with those knowledgeable in the use of diet drugs.

As a general principle, I am opposed to the use of drugs for dieting, but I know there are qualified health professionals who do not share my opinion. If you anticipate using dieting drugs, I hope it would be for a short term only to get started and that you would soon develop the kind of behavioral and diet changes that would allow you to successfully manage your weight.

3. DAILY ACTIVITIES: As I have repeatedly stated, there may not be anything more important to you from the standpoint of physical fitness, health, and weight control than an active lifestyle.

Ninety-four Ways, Tricks, Reasons, and Thoughts to Lose Weight*

1. Don't waste your time and money on fad diets, diet pills, or magic potions that promise weight loss overnight. Most of the weight you lose on these is from water, not fat.

2. Keep records of how much you eat, when and where you eat, what you're doing while you eat, who you're eating with, and your mood. After a week or two, go over your records and look for any patterns that occur when you overeat.

3. Do you have any eating behaviors you would like to change—such as eating when you're upset? Try changing just one habit at a time. Don't tackle another until you're sure you have the first one under control.

4. Store everything you eat in the kitchen. Don't keep any food in your car, desk, or nightstand.

5. Start to measure or weigh all your food portions so you know exactly how much food you're eating.

6. Eat your meals at the same time each day. That way, you condition your body to expect food at certain times.

7. Eat breakfast. People who skip breakfast are more likely to binge later in the day.

8. Chew gum to prevent nibbling while cooking.

9. Don't snack while watching television or reading. You could easily consume an entire bag of potato chips without being aware of it.

10. Drink a glass of water before you eat—it will help make your stomach feel fuller.

11. Eat slowly, and put your fork down after every bite. Make each meal last 15 to 20 minutes.

12. Don't shovel food into your mouth. Taste and enjoy each mouthful.

13. If you're having trouble eating slowly, try eating with chopsticks or with the fork in the wrong hand.

14. Eat off a small plate. It makes small portions look like more.

15. Remove serving bowls and plates of food from the table while eating. They may tempt you into eating more than you really want.

16. Wait 20 minutes before having a second helping. It usually takes that long for your stomach to tell your brain that you're full.

17. Always leave a bite of food on your plate. It's better to let food go to waste than to your waist. Save leftovers for another meal.

18. When you begin to feel full, try this exercise: place your hands firmly on the edge of the table. Then straighten your arms while moving your torso away from the table. Stand up and walk away.

19. Stay busy doing things you enjoy. Some people eat when they're bored.

20. Try to get at least 20 to 30 minutes of exercise a day. How about a daily routine of walking, jogging, or aerobics in time to your favorite music?

21. Exercise along with an exercise program on television or an exercise video.

22. Sign up for an activity or exercise class (such as volleyball or aerobics). With a little companionship and some friendly competition, exercise can seem more like fun than work.

*1-50 are from the American Dairy Society.

23. Don't worry; exercise won't increase your appetite. In fact, some people find they aren't as hungry after a good workout.

24. Walk or ride your bicycle to the store, post office, or library. Walking just once around the block each day, you could lose over 5 pounds in a year.

25. Kill two birds with one stone. Burn up calories while working around the house. You can use up 100 calories by cleaning for a half hour or mowing the lawn for 17 minutes.

26. Use the stairs at work or at the mall instead of using the elevator or escalator.

27. While no single food is fattening, too much of anything can be. Your body will turn 3,500 calories of unused energy into 1 pound of fat, regardless of whether those calories come from cookies or celery.

28. Replace fruit canned in heavy syrup with fresh fruit or with fruit canned in water or its own juices. Compare the calories in one cup of peaches:
- Canned in water—58
- Fresh—73
- Canned in juice—109
- Canned in light syrup—136
- Canned in heavy syrup—190

29. Many people watching their weight drink low-fat 2 percent milk, low-fat 1 percent milk, skim milk, or buttermilk.

30. Did you know that just two tablespoons of French dressing add 134 calories to your low-calorie salad? Try lemon juice or reduced-calorie dressings on your salads instead.

31. Buy lean cuts of meat, and trim off all visible fat.

32. Pass up the skin on that piece of chicken. Better yet, remove the skin before cooking. That way there will be less fat and fewer calories.

33. Eat fewer fried foods. Frying can triple the number of calories in foods. Look at what it does to a half cup of potatoes:
- Boiled—67 calories
- Hash-browned—163 calories
- French-fried—180 calories

34. You don't have to give up all your favorite foods—just eat smaller portions. Have two slices of pizza instead of three. Or share dessert with a friend.

35. Buy chips, candy, and other snacks in small individual-size packages. That way you'll have built-in portion control.

36. When you buy or bake a cake, slice it into individual pieces, and freeze the pieces separately. This makes it harder for you to eat unconsciously.

37. If you're absolutely famished and it's not mealtime, set a timer for 20 minutes. If you're still hungry after 20 minutes, go ahead and have a nutritious snack.

38. Keep nutrient-rich snacks on hand. The following snacks have 100 calories or fewer:
- ½ cup chocolate milk
- 1 medium apple, orange, or pear
- 1 oz. stick of string cheese
- 1 slice whole wheat toast and butter
- 1 cup light yogurt
- ½ cup mushrooms, ½ cup cucumbers, ½ cup salsa

- ¼ cup pumpkin seeds
- 3 oz. frozen yogurt

39. Store low-calorie snacks in the front of your refrigerator or cabinets—so you see them first.

40. Make snacking an effort. Buy snack foods that require some work, such as unpopped popcorn or an orange that needs peeling.

41. Brush your teeth after every meal. Sometimes that can be enough to discourage between-meal snacking.

42. Plan ahead. If you know you're going to a party or a big dinner, cut back on your caloric intake earlier in the day.

43. If you do overeat, don't give up. The most you'll gain is a pound or so. Get back to your eating plan as soon as possible.

44. Praise yourself every day! Give yourself a pat on the back for getting some exercise or following your eating plan. Especially on days when you weren't "perfect," find something you did right—and compliment yourself for that.

45. Weigh yourself no more than once a week, at the same time of day. Your weight goes up and down from day to day, so it might be misleading (and possibly discouraging) to weigh yourself too often.

46. Pay attention to how your clothes fit. When they feel looser, you know you're losing fat. Congratulations!

47. Keep records of your weight and measurements. A graph will give you an even better picture of your losses.

48. Generally, the more slowly you take the weight off, the longer you keep it off. Aim for a weight loss of ½ to 1 pound a week. Remember, 3,500 fewer calories per week (500 calories a day) can result in a 1-pound weight loss in a week.

49. When you lose weight, have your clothes taken in, or give them away. If you gain a few pounds, your smaller-sized wardrobe will give you instant feedback that you need to exercise more or eat a little less.

50. Reinforce success. Reward yourself for each five-pound weight loss with a little treat—a tape or a compact disc, a manicure, a new book, or a ticket to the theater.

51. A large amount of exercise is not necessary to burn up enough calories to be effective. Any exercise is better than no exercise.

52. Answer the phone that is farthest away.

53. Use the rest room that is farthest away.

54. Stand instead of sit; sit instead of lying down whenever possible.

55. Walk to children's rooms to talk to them instead of raising your voice to be heard.

56. Take articles upstairs several times throughout the day rather than piling things on the steps for a later trip.

57. Walk to work, or start your walking part way and increase the distance.

58. Get off the bus a few blocks early, or arrange to park your car farther away.

59. Stand up and move around occasionally.

60. Fidget and shake your legs. You can burn up several hundred calories a day by constant motion.

61. Choose physical activities that fit your schedule, likes, and budget. If you prefer an exercise group or doing your exercise at home, be sure to choose carefully. Do what you enjoy and what will keep you coming back.

62. Find a partner, someone to encourage you and hold you accountable.

63. Remember that low-fat or nonfat foods still have calories and that any extra calories consumed that are not burned off will end up as extra fat.

64. Remember that it is unwise for a man to reduce his calories to below 1,500 to 1,600 a day and for a woman to reduce her calories to below 1,000 to 1,200 calories a day. While on these restricted diets, you probably will want to take some vitamin and nutritional supplements.

65. You can't eliminate all fat from your diet, nor should you. We all need some fat. It is an essential nutrient just like protein and carbohydrates.

66. Post the food pyramid on your refrigerator or some obvious location. Remember that serving sizes usually tend to be too large.

67. Avoid very low-calorie weight loss diets such as liquid diets.

68. Don't buy the myth that just because you are getting older you should be putting weight on. Skinny people die at the slowest rates.

69. Don't accept the myth "I'll never lose enough weight to improve my health." Losing even a few pounds helps. For example, if you drop your weight 2 pounds, on the average your cholesterol drops three points. Normal-weight people are much more apt to have normal blood pressure, whereas overweight people are much more apt to have high blood pressure.

70. Not all calories are created equal. The calories from fatty foods are more likely to make you fat than calories from carbohydrates or proteins.

71. Losing weight is not the hard part—keeping it off is, so make the necessary lifestyle changes and behavioral changes you need to maintain your weight loss.

72. You cannot target one area of fat only. Exercise and diet can melt away fat, but you can't target specific areas.

73. Don't use emotional stress as an excuse to eat. Find other creative ways to release emotional stress other than deliberate emotional eating.

74. Love yourself. Decide to lose excess weight because you are a wonderful person, not in order to become one.

75. Choose an eating plan you can live with.

76. Pump up the produce. Remember the Garden of Eden concept. If it was grown there, it is probably good to eat and good for you.

77. Think fruit for dessert.

78. Keep homemade frozen fruit juice bars in the freezer.

79. Stock your refrigerator with cut-up fruits and veggies for easy munching.

80. Make up creative excuses to exercise.

81. Take a walk or get some other exercise whenever you feel stressed.

82. Go outside to play at least once a week.

83. Don't rely on drugs for your ticket to success.

84. Dump the diet; go on a *food plan*.

85. Avoid skipping meals. You may get too ravenously hungry if you do that and thus will be likely to overeat at your next meal.

86. Disarm cravings with the "five Ds" (taken from Marsha Hudnall's *Low Calorie Recipes*):

Delay at least 10 minutes before you eat so that your action is conscious, not impulsive.

Distract yourself by engaging in an activity that is incompatible with eating, such as riding your bicycle or mowing the lawn.

Distance yourself from the food—leave the room; ask the waiter to remove your plate; don't park at the food court entrance to the mall.

Determine how important it really is for you to eat the food and how much you really want it.

Decide what amount is reasonable and appropriate; then eat it slowly and enjoy.

87. Don't choose fasting for anything greater than a few hours and certainly not more than a single day.

88. Avoid skin patches, food scams, and other fad and too-good-to-be-true diets.

89. Don't be afraid to join a reputable weight loss program. There are many excellent ones out there that will give you built-in accountability and camaraderie, a very important process in your life.

90. You do not have to stop eating red meat, but make sure you take lean cuts and smaller servings.

91. Supplementing your food plan with vitamin pills is probably a very reasonable plan.

92. Do not use body wraps, sauna rooms, and so on to lose weight. The only thing you do by these techniques is lose fluid.

93. Learn to love and accept yourself as you are, and realize that no matter what your weight, you are a wonderful, beautiful person created by God.

94. Remember: diets don't make you beautiful. Beauty certainly is far more than skin deep and is principally inward graces, strength, and good qualities.

> **We are in the era of self-induced premature deaths. The top three causes of premature death are tobacco, poor diet and inactivity, and alcohol. The top nine causes of premature death are all self-controlled.**
>
> —C. Everett Koop

DIET, EXERCISE, AND WEIGHT LOSS

An article in the January 1997 issue of *Runners World* reports,

> If you want to lose weight, you have three options. You can (1) go on a diet, (2) exercise more, or (3) do some combination of the two. Researchers at Baylor College of Medicine in Houston re-

cently tested each of these weight-loss methods on obese subjects to see which worked best over the long term. The winner: exercise.

The dieters followed a well-balanced, low-cholesterol diet made up of 30 percent fat, 50 percent carbohydrates, and 20 percent protein. The exercisers walked vigorously for at least 45 minutes three to five days a week. The diet-plus-exercise group followed both regimens.

At the end of the first year, the diet-plus-exercise group had lost the most weight. Next were the dieters, who lost nearly as much weight. The exercisers came in last with the least amount of weight loss.

However, after 24 months and the dust had settled, the study was over, and the monitoring done, the exercisers had maintained the best weight loss reduction while the others had returned to near prestudy level.

DOES GOD CARE IF I AM OVERWEIGHT?

It has been said that we would be a kinder and happier society if we were all blind. The Scriptures clearly tell us that people look on the outward appearances but God looks on the heart. With God there is no race, gender, size, talent, or social discrimination.

God obviously loves variety. He did not intend that we would all be similar in appearance. His template for the human body was not the 5'10", thin, female model or the 6'2" muscular bodybuilder. However, since our bodies are the temples of the Holy Spirit, it stands to reason that we should do our part to provide a fit and healthy dwelling place for our God.

DOCTOR'S ORDERS: RX FOR WEIGHT LOSS

▶ Eat right, and remember that *fat is fattening.*

▶ Develop habits that are constructive and healthful, for *habits make it happen.*

▶ Exercise faithfully for *exercise is essential.*

Do all the good you can,
By all the means you can,
In all the ways you can,
In all the places you can,
In all the times you can,
To all the people you can,
As long as ever you can!

—John Wesley's
"Rule for Christian Living"

CHAPTER 13

A WORD FROM THE PROFESSOR . . .
GENEROSITY

A small study in east Denver, a Sunday afternoon in the mid-1960s, and the four New Testament Gospels provided the context for my choice to become a professional social worker. That afternoon changed me forever. From that day forward I became a "dually diagnosed" person, that is, both a clergyman and a social worker. In the mid-'60s I determined to invest much of my energy to wholistic ministries.

Now, some 30 years later, I reflect. Did that afternoon make any difference? For me? For my denomination? For my students? When the Holy Spirit led me to begin a reorganization of my career and life, I was called to serve others within the upheavals and the pressing human needs of my society. It was and is a mandate.

GENEROSITY AND SELFISHNESS

Dick Cavalli, creator of the cartoon strip *Winthrop*, gives us insight into the human condition. In one strip Winthrop's buddy announces, "If

I could have three wishes, I'd wish for all the money in the world, and all the candy in the world, and I'd wish for three more wishes." As they parted, Winthrop mumbled, "It isn't every day you get to see such a perfect example of pure naked greed."

The *Idaho Press-Tribune* reports a lesson of another kind. The newspaper ran a story on January 29, 1982, during a period of high unemployment, about Ben Gaman, a single 27-year-old machinist for Pratt and Whitney Aircraft. Gaman voluntarily sacrificed his job so a union man with less seniority who had a pregnant wife and two small children would not be laid off. The married man said, "I'm shocked, because I can't believe there's a person with a heart like that. People like him are hard to come by."

GENEROSITY: A REDISCOVERY OF SOCIETY'S SOUL

Compassionate generosity, as a lifestyle, is a bone that gets caught sideways in the throat of our modern society. Senator Bill Armstrong of Colorado is purported to have said, "Our national motto is no longer 'In God we trust,' but 'Every man for himself.'"

Meg Greenfield wrote an essay in the November 16, 1987, edition of *Newsweek* about "our affliction with greed," or "the Me Age," in which she stated, "Even our altruism is self-indulgent, greedy. How many of these crusades for one deprived group or another have we seen picked up, exploited, and dropped as its 'feel good' potential is used up and those allegedly giving their all have no more to get from the crusade in the way of personal gratification?"

The same point of view is emphasized by Karl Olsson in the June 1973 issue of *Faith at Work* as he describes "the bad Samaritan":

> What is it then to be a bad Samaritan? I believe it is to help people largely out of my own need. It is to give assistance because I am guilty and need to atone or because benefaction has such a high social value. To be a bad Samaritan is to ignore the real needs of the other person or to assume hastily that I know what they are. To be a bad Samaritan is also to generalize about need and about prescription. It is the besetting need of social machinery which does not have the time or the interest to look at persons. It operates with a handful of diagnoses and a handful of prescriptions.

Authentic generosity gets us in touch with our true and best selves. It draws us to a God of grace and mercy. Generosity is an admission that life is a shared enterprise with others. Compassion that yields generous actions with one's time, money, resources, and talents becomes especially significant in our needy society.

SERVING JESUS BY SERVING OTHERS

Mother Teresa and her sisters, the Missionaries of Charity, have proven that the stubborn and tireless energy of a dedicated few can redefine the meaning of compassion for an entire generation. What compelled an 18-year-old school girl from a close-knit family to leave the protection of home to go to India to become a nun? What forces later led that same diminutive person to leave the shelter of the cloister and Loreto School to move into the slums of Calcutta?

Mother Teresa spoke of her departure from the Loreto convent with its pleasant gardens, eager school girls, and rewarding academic appointments to live among the poorest of the poor as a "call within a call." Malcomb Muggeridge contrasts his response to Calcutta's poor with the deliberate choice made by Mother Teresa. He writes:

> I ran away and stayed away; Mother Teresa moved in and stayed. She, a nun, rather slightly built, with a few rupees in her pocket; not particularly clever, or particularly gifted in the art of persuasion. Just with this Christian love shining about her; in her heart and on her lips. Just prepared to follow her Lord, and in accord with his instructions to regard every derelict left to die in the streets as him; to hear in the cry of every abandoned child, even in the tiny squeak of [a] discarded fetus, the cry of the Bethlehem child; to recognize in every leper's stumps the hands that once touched sightless eyes and made them see, rested on distracted heads and made them calm, brought back health to sick flesh and twisted limbs.

Mother Teresa stepped outside the routine and invested herself with compassionate generosity. She recognized the Lord Christ in each person she served. Muggeridge describes this new spiritual level of awareness:

An awareness that these dying and derelict men and women, these lepers with stumps instead of hands, these unwanted children, were not pitiable, repulsive or forlorn, but rather dear and delightful; as it might be, friends of long standing, brothers and sisters. How is it to be explained—the very heart and mystery of the Christian faith? To sooth those battered old heads, to grasp those poor stumps, to take in one's arms those children consigned to dustbins, because it is his head, as they are his stumps and his children, of whom it was said that whosoever received one child in his name received him.

SHARING OUR RESOURCES

The act of experiencing compassion for the hurting, messy, and unattractive members of the human race is called identification. Genuine compassion moves beyond pity or sympathy. Compassion begins with the acknowledgement that all persons have value, worth, and dignity. All persons, regardless of how boring, brutish, bad, and barren of merit, deserve opportunity, acceptance, and love.

The incarnation of Christ—God moving in among us as one of us—forever changed the meaning of identification. This amazing theological truth is perhaps best understood as we get glimpses of it in the lives of people.

Francis was one of those people. Theologian and educator Michael Christensen writes about this saint's deepening identification with God as Creator.

In 1182 Giovanni Francesco Bernardone was born into the home of a wealthy textile merchant in the town of Assisi, Italy. As a young man, he spent a year as a prisoner of war and then experienced a lengthy debilitating illness. During and after these two traumatic periods, Francis began to see and understand a new relationship with all of nature. He learned to recognize God in creation and saw himself as related to every living thing.

It was at his point of connection with God and creation that Francis of Assisi would make the reckless identification of himself with all creatures, regardless. Christensen captures the pivotal point of Francis becoming "the saint from Assisi." He wrote:

As a young man, Francis had a particular distaste for lepers. While riding horseback one fine day, he encountered a leper
standing beside the road. Initially repulsed, then feeling a strong
surge of compassion, Francis dismounted and put some money
into the man's hands. "More is required of you," said a still small
voice in Francis' heart. In a dramatic gesture he would later regard as a turning point in his life, Francis kissed the leper. From
that time on he gave away everything he owned and began to see
himself as having a special bond with the poor and disadvantaged.

Is it any wonder that more has been written about Francis than any
other saint? Francis of Assisi was canonized within two years following
his death. A special order of Christian ministry, the Franciscans, was organized around the memory and the ministry modeled by Francis. A
statue of Francis stands over the California city named after him, San
Francisco. And one won't spend many months around a community of
worshiping believers before hearing someone sing from the prayer of
Francis.

Lord, make me an instrument of Thy peace:
Where there is hatred, let me sow love;

The closing lines recall this man who moved in among the poor
and have-nots and identified with them:

For it is in giving that we receive;

. . . .

It is in dying that we are born to eternal life!

Christian love, then, is not simply warm feelings. It is not simply
the proper organization of words into phrases of inspiration. Genuine
Christian love produces generosity that gets mixed in with all the
mess and meanness of the everyday world. It addresses the needs at
hand in the name of Jesus.

"Love is not primarily a feeling," George Lyons notes, "nor even
a disposition; it is active goodwill, seeking what is in the long-term
best interests of the other."

Franco builds on the theme of compassionate generosity. He observed, "We cannot love without getting dirty. We cannot love at a distance. . . . We cannot love by proxy. We cannot serve through our min-

isters. We cannot heal wounds through our missionaries. Not possibly, not ever! You and I have got to be involved with somebody."

BECOMING A PERSON OF GENEROSITY

Do we dare become persons of compassionate generosity? Where do we begin? Perhaps an old story applies here. A tourist interrupted an old Irish farmer by asking, "Tell me, sir, how might I find my way to Dublin?" The farmer responded, "If I were going to Dublin, I wouldn't start from here." If we become persons of generosity, we must begin here, now, and with what we have.

THE PROF'S HOMEWORK ASSIGNMENT: GIVING ALL WE CAN

At the beginning of this chapter you saw John Wesley's "Rule for Christian Living." Wesley appropriately noted that doing good is about a multiplicity of opportunities for our entire lives. Money is a flagship that sets the direction for other segments of life. In 1748 Wesley preached a sermon titled "The Use of Money." Here are his points:

1. "Gain all you can."
2. "Save all you can."
3. "Give all you can."

Reflect on Wesley's points. What does the audit of my checkbook tell me about my generosity? What changes do I wish to make?

Wesley practiced what he preached. He claimed that if he left more than 10 pounds in his will when he died that he justifiably could be called a thief. The record shows that he left only some loose money in his clothes and bureau and 6 pounds for the poor men who were to carry his body to the grave. It is estimated that Wesley gave some 30,000 pounds to charity during his lifetime. He believed Paul's admonition to Timothy: "We brought nothing into the world, and we can take nothing out of it" (1 Tim. 6:7).

If a man cleanses himself from the [ignoble], he will be
an instrument for noble purposes, made holy, useful to
the Master and prepared to do any good work.

—2 Tim. 2:21

CHAPTER 14

A WORD FROM THE PROFESSOR . . .
WORK

arry and I trapped gophers for E. R. Knott as our first away-from-home job. Mr. Knott owned and operated the farm immediately north of our place. He paid us 25 cents for every gopher tail we delivered. We didn't get rich, but this job fostered the development of a strong work ethic.

We learned that daily monitoring of the traps produced more bounty than haphazard attention. We grasped the connection between effort, productivity, and income. Also, we discovered that outside factors (like Mr. Knott's irrigation schedule) sometimes interfere with even our best efforts.

Later we hired out to load hay bales on the Jacksons' farm, hoe beets for the Scotts, and drive trucks for Morey's Custom Hay Services. During the summer of 1954, prior to our junior year in high school, we virtually ran (from our perspective) the large alfalfa farm of Hayward Jack. By the time we were 18 we were confirmed believers in the American work ethic. We understood work and godliness as compatible and related matters.

We all have 168 hours each week to spend as we wish. In modern Western societies most adults invest almost one-third of each week's hours in matters pertaining to work. The self-employed, professionals, and many hourly wage earners spend 50 or more hours per week working, preparing for work, and commuting to and from work. An activity that usurps one-third of our time deserves careful scrutiny. Any discussion of wholeness must consider this segment of our lives.

WHY WORK?

An assortment of *whys* haunt us while on the job. Why work in this job, for this company, with these people?

These recurring *whys* push us back to the larger "Why work?" question. My social work students enjoy grappling with the question of why work is important for modern Americans. Each year the students generate a host of reasons, including to earn money, to gain social status, to occupy time, to achieve a personal identity, to find a source of meaning, and so on. Let's consider the biblical basis for work and the societal rationale.

Why Work? A Biblical Basis

The Creator God modeled work. God was the first self-employed Worker. He first worked spans of time we call the days of creation. Humans, God's final act of creation, were assigned work from the beginning. We often identify work with the Fall, humanity's engagement with sin. Wrong. Human work began in the beautiful garden of God's handiwork prior to the Fall. Hear the record:

> The LORD God took the man and put him in the Garden of Eden to work it and take care of it. . . . He brought them [the animals] to the man to see what he would name them; and whatever the man called each living creature, that was its name *(Gen. 2:15, 19)*.

As a child during the 1940s and 1950s, I accepted the witness of the American church that we are workers together with God (see 1 Cor. 3:9). The church taught me that Christian living is 24 hours a day, 7 days a week, 365 days a year, for a lifetime. Thus, it made sense to me that our family stopped every morning, immediately following breakfast, for family devotions. In this religious ceremony we prayed for God's grace and strength for the work of the day, wherever it occurred—school, kitchen, barn, or field. It seemed to me that work was included in the Westminster Shorter Catechism's statement about the chief goal of human life. It declared that humanity's main purpose is "to glorify God, and to enjoy Him forever." Giving glory to God included, in my thinking, all day every day. Thus, early in life I sensed that while I was pitching hay and milking cows, I was engaged in God's work.

Theologians teach us that humans are the *imago Dei* (the image of God) in the whole of the created order. We have been given the responsibility of representing the Creator God in His creation. We, then, are colaborers with God. In the July 29, 1977, issue of *Christianity Today*, New Testament scholar W. Ward Gasque noted this coworker assignment: "In more everyday terms, this means that God is concerned as much with a person's work as with his worship. . . . Work can never degenerate to meaningless drudgery but will always be permeated by a sense of divine purpose. In one's daily work, even if it seems insignificant, one is involved in the service of God and man, seeking to bring glory to God."

Martin Luther observed, "A housemaid who does her work is no farther away from God than the priest in the pulpit." Truly, our work is a call to worship.

Why Work? For the Well-being of Society

We have already said that Americans are interdependent. Each of us has his or her own "end of society's log" to carry. If for some reason I cannot carry my end of the log, then society is less productive. Under these arrangements I become *dependent* and thus must ask other persons to help with my responsibilities.

We don't expect all people to be productive and involved in the world of work. We permit children to be dependent. We permit frail elderly to be dependent. We permit certain categories of the disabled and mentally ill to be dependent. In other cases, such as in the criminal justice system, we force some persons to be dependent upon society. For the most part, however, the majority of us need to log our time in the workforce from age 18 through 65.

We have a tall order, then, to make sure today's children will be employable when they reach age 18. This responsibility includes provision for proper nutrition, safe environments, high-quality education, necessary health care, appropriate socialization, and real access to opportunity. Those who don't have these benefits will be unable, as a rule, to become productive workers.

WHICH JOB SHALL I CHOOSE?

Is there a "right" job or career for each of us? Does God have a blueprint room where He keeps a life plan for all of us? Should each of us expect a special calling so that a choice of a career is as conspicuous and easy to read as a street sign? The dramatic call of God upon Paul, who was struck by a bright light, is the exception, not the rule.

Most Christians simply "stumble" into their employment. It is a combination of timing, location, contacts, previous experiences, and the peculiar characteristics of the surrounding labor market. For a Christian these factors are mixed with faith in God and what we understand we must do in order to serve our generation.

We twin brothers came by our careers by dramatically different routes. Larry was captured early by the wonders of medical practice and was never deterred from that choice. I long planned to be a journalist. One summer morning in 1954 a radical change of direction occurred. God did not knock me to the ground, as He did the apostle Paul. Instead, He found me driving a tractor with a hay wagon in tow. The remainder of the morning was an intense ongoing interaction with God as I abandoned other goals and agreed to work in professional ministry within the church.

I am the first to argue, however, that my work has not been more "Christian" than Larry's work—simply different. I have received a paycheck each month from a bank account held by the church. Larry, a self-employed medical practitioner, signs his own salary checks. We both, however, have been engaged in Christian ministry. This is so because Christian ministry is determined by allegiance to Christ whereby each of us offers daily (continuously with every breath) the totality of our life, including our vocation. The apostle Paul captured the sense of this way of looking at one's vocation as he wrote:

> In view of God's mercy, give yourselves as daily offerings to God. Make these offerings holy and pleasing to God as a form of continuous worship. Do not conform any longer to the pattern of this secular world, but be transformed so that you seek to do what is good and God's will (*Rom. 12:1-2, author's paraphrase*).

This approach defines life, in all of its dimensions, as a gift offered to the Holy God. In this sense, work is not something I do; rather, work is part of this wholeness of me that I offer as a gift of love, obedience, and praise to God. In his letter to the Colossian Christians, Paul picks up the theme of Christian work with these statements:

> And whatever you do, whether in word or deed, do it all in the name of the Lord Jesus, giving thanks to God the Father through him. . . . Whatever you do, work at it with all your heart, as working for the Lord, not for men *(Col. 3:17, 23)*.

WHAT KIND OF WORKER SHALL I BE?

The best worker I can be is the only suitable choice. What indicators guide us to be workers of quality and excellence? From an employee's first week in the labor force, we all know that hiring a person, assigning a job title, and designating a workstation does not guarantee quality. People bring varying degrees of readiness, commitment, motivation, personal disciplines, and imagination to their jobs.

A Christian worker displays the qualities of character, competence, cooperation, and confidence.

Character

What kind of person am I? A person of character, among other things, is an individual of honesty, genuineness, fairness, depth, firmly held principles, empathy, sensitivity, and accountability. A person of character is motivated from the inside out. He or she is sensitive to external contexts but not controlled by pressure from the outside. The person of character has an internal sense of who he or she is and what he or she needs to be and do.

Character is not something we put on and take off as convenient. Character seeps out through our conversation, our actions, our relationships, our allocations of time, and the spirit of person we project to others around us. Our true character comes out in the experiences of life, especially in the workplace.

Competence

Some decades ago I earned several academic degrees and gained some much-desired professional credentials. These add strength to my résumé and cover some otherwise empty spaces on my office wall. These long-ago achievements, however, don't guarantee ongoing competence. Competency is ongoing and continuing. I must read new literature and review new methods and models of social work practice.

Each year I submit a "professional development plan." Part of the process is a self-assessment of how well I met the professional development plan of the previous year. A serious gap between projections and achievements requires explanation.

Cooperation

Teamwork is a critical element of excellence. Teamwork leads to an appropriate sense of both humility and humor about ourselves. Often I need to recognize that the weight of the world does not rest upon my shoulders. This reminder is a great relief. When I am weary to the bone because of long hours of work, I find it necessary to admit that the college, the city, and the world will get along quite well after I'm dead and gone. In fact, I've requested my campus colleagues to wait 10 minutes after I die before they begin discussing a replacement for my position. I doubt I'll get the full 10 minutes of silence and respect, but it's fun to pretend.

Imagine how much good could be accomplished if no one cared about who received the credit. We shouldn't be faceless and nameless cogs at our workplaces, but most of us need a new level of appreciation for our coworkers. We're team members. Synergy suggests that the whole is more than the total of the separate parts. Synergy calls for us to work together so that we might accomplish more than each of us could achieve separately.

Confidence

Confidence, as used here, refers to how others regard my work. It is not a mood or a state of poise by which I go about an activity. Confidence is a status both earned and assigned day by day by work colleagues, supervisors, customers, consumers, and clients. I cannot dictate that any of the above categories of persons must regard my work positively. Somehow in a predictable but not easily explained dynamic, confidence is either granted or withheld. It springs out of the mix of character, competence, and cooperation discussed above. If I am a person of character, competence, and cooperation, I may expect others to place confidence in me and my performance.

WORK IS PART OF THE WHOLE

Everything we Christians do must be filtered through the standard "Is this acceptable to God and a way to serve God?" Thus, the totality of life for each unfolding moment is offered as a gift to Jesus Christ. How we use our time, the ways we spend our dollars, our choices of relationships, and the careers we enter are all matters of prayer. We desire that everything about us be pleasing to God.

Recently David Blowers, career Christian missionary to Haiti, spoke about the psalmist's phrase "establish the work of our hands" (Ps. 90:17). David is a skilled carpenter and helps Haitian congregations build chapels and schools. He told about doing work in a remote mountain village of Haiti. The first day there he was awakened before dawn by the voice of his host, a Haitian pastor, praying aloud. In the course of the prayer, he submitted his family, his congregation, and David (specifically by name) into God's hands. David found profound confirmation about his own work during the emerging light of that new day. "The work we do becomes God's work when we put it in His hands," he observed. David's words summarize well the connection of work and wholeness.

THE PROFESSOR'S HOMEWORK ASSIGNMENT

Reflect on the following questions, or discuss them with a Christian friend:

▶ Is my career (job) a valuable investment of God's gift of time to me?

▶ How is society in general or persons in particular benefited by my work?

▶ Are any persons or groups of people exploited by my work?

▶ Is the product or service produced by my work a worthy extension of who I am as a person? Do I feel good about the product I produce through my work so I can say proudly, "This is me"?

▶ Is my work a way of bringing honor and glory to God, and a witness to others about the God I serve?

A FINAL WORD FROM THE DOCTOR . . .
ENCORE

They came to my office on the very same day.

She was a 41-year-old mother of three who, in the course of the examination, was asked to hop first on one foot and then on the other. Her excess weight, weak muscles, and total lack of confidence prevented her from getting off the floor. She couldn't even jump half an inch.

He was a 46-year-old middle-echelon bank officer with the proverbial paunch and aching back. Out of shape, he was at a high risk of heart disease and knew it. He felt rotten and wasn't doing anything about it.

I observed that the self-esteem of these two had been effectively obliterated. They believed they were unable to do anything about their predicaments. They had no zest or optimism in their lives. It was depressing to be around them.

These two people are not unique. Many of my patients are in a similar predicament. Their physical complaints range from lack of energy to being 150 pounds overweight with chronic knee, back, or joint problems. Personally and professionally, their lives range from ho-hum to total disaster, and they feel helpless to do anything about it.

TWO FRIENDS: INCH-BY-INCH SUICIDE

Bob was an outstanding, well-known, contributing member of my community and church. He had a successful law practice and many community interests. He was a gifted communicator and a sensitive, loving father and husband. He was a growing person with the best days of his life ahead.

One day while he was working on his boat, he had a heart attack and died without warning or fanfare. He was 52 years old with no known previous heart disease. He left behind a lovely wife and two daughters.

Ed was a special friend and colleague of mine. As a pediatrician he was a warm, loving servant of humanity. He was competent and successful, committed to his patients, community, church, and family. Ed had a known heart condition. Despite this, he continued to be overweight and underfit. Then it happened. One cool, rainy day while cleaning the gutters of his house, he died. He was 53 years old. He left behind a lovely wife, wonderful children, a needy community, and the best years of his life.

My friends' death certificates read basically the same: "advanced coronary artery disease" By all rights, the death certificates could have read "suicide."

Yes, suicide—inch by inch. It wasn't suicide by design. They didn't pick a place and leave a note. Instead, they chose a *fatal lifestyle*. For whatever reasons, they chose the uninformed, easy way.

You've heard about my two patients and two friends. Now I'll tell you about me.

HEART DISEASE AT AGE 35

At 35 years of age, I had just completed 26 years of school and training. I was about to set up a practice as the pioneer orthopaedic surgeon in a lovely community. Youth, training, work ethic, and a high energy level, all pointed to sure success. Everything was going my way.

Being my always-in-a-hurry self, I was running a half block to my car to save time. Suddenly I felt my heart go berserk. My heart's timing mechanism had faltered, resulting in an arrhythmia (rapid, irregular, and ineffective heart beats). In my confusion and panic, the first words that came to my mind were my mother's: "Larry, if you don't slow down and take care of yourself, you'll have a heart attack by the time you're 35!"

I felt as though my future had been maliciously attacked. In the hospital bed I pondered my plans and goals. They might go unrealized. I thought about my young wife, who shared my dreams and worked so hard to help me achieve them. And what about my young son and younger daughters? Would they be able to get along without me? Would I be deprived of an opportunity to laugh with them, to share in their joys and successes? Would I be there to help carry their loads in times of pain and struggle? Who would take my place in the work of the Kingdom at church and in the community?

Fortunately, treatment was successful, and medication controlled the problem.

In time I forgot what I had so abruptly learned. I forgot about the medication. I forgot about getting enough rest and relief from stress. I forgot about eating a prudent diet. I forgot about exercise. I was back to being my striving, driving, hard-working, achieving, important self. Responsibilities in the office, church, and community continued to grow. I now had five children, two of them very young.

Potential disaster struck again.

I was running the half block from my office to the hospital when the same sequence started all over. The same symptoms, the same fears, and the same treatments.

Once again, treatment was successful. But this time, I realized I was in a predicament. I was 42 years old with a history of heart disease. I led a high-stress, overworked existence. I was completely out of shape. Life insurance companies considered me a high risk. The increased insurance costs didn't bother me nearly as much as knowing that *they knew* I was a much higher death risk than other men my age.

I decided to beat the odds. I took the challenge of creating a healthy lifestyle.

I'll never forget the first day I donned my sneakers and walked/ jogged a mile. It took me about 10 minutes, and I felt as if I were dying. But I kept at it.

Things have changed since then. I'm wearing out my 10th pair of real running shoes. I'm able to run 10 miles at a faster pace and with much greater ease than that first mile 13 years ago. I have learned to enjoy a diet that is good for me (low in fats and cholesterol and higher in fiber and nutrients). I have fun competing in 10,000-meter runs, taking long bicycle tours, and playing sports with my children. The maximum-stress treadmill test (the state-of-the-art fitness evaluation) places me in the "excellent" category for my age group. Today I am happier. I am a more creative physician and surgeon. But more than all of that, I am adding years to my life and energy to my days so I can love and serve where God has placed me. My wholeness journey needed physical fitness and physical discipline to be more complete.

Your Story: Is Your Lifestyle Suicidal?

What is your story? Where are you on your health and wholeness journey? Most of you are no doubt in the "I never really thought that much about it" category. Some of you are in the "I've started a physical fitness or self-improvement program" group. A lot of you have quieted that inner voice of conscience by telling yourselves, "I'm going to get in shape as soon as . . ." Whatever your status, you need to be aware of some of the chilling realities of poor choices.

As a quick evaluation of your level of fitness, ask yourself these helpful, if not all scientific, questions:

1. Do you weigh more than you did at age 20?
2. Women, has your dress size increased since age 20? Men, have you let your belt out several inches since that age?
3. Is your resting heart rate above 75 beats per minute? (Resting heart rate is how many times your heart beats for one minute while you are at rest.)
4. Can you pinch more than an inch (waist)?
5. Do you dislike what you see when you stand nude in front of a full-length mirror?
6. Do you get short of breath after two flights of stairs?
7. Do you eat whatever you like, without counting calories, reading labels, or avoiding excess fats and cholesterol?
8. Finally, have you failed to establish a course of action that will take you where you want to be physically, intellectually, and spiritually?

"If you continue doing what you're doing, you'll get more of what you've got." Do you like what you've got?

The purpose of this book is to help you live better and longer. Better, because it doesn't make much sense to squeak a few more years into a dull and meaningless existence. If we are Christians fulfilling God's purposes here on earth, we are needed. We are important. We have a unique opportunity to make a difference. Longer, because it is a proven fact that physically fit, socially competent, and spiritually alive people are healthier, happier, and more productive.

Back to my two friends. If Bob and Ed were alive today, would our world be a better place? Absolutely. Their influence was important.

And me? What would my life be like today if I hadn't changed my bad habits? I certainly wouldn't be enjoying the lifestyle I now have.

My two patients? They've been in and out of my office several times. They have yet to follow through on my instructions for physical fitness. Sometimes they're better, sometimes worse. They'll probably die prematurely, and in the meantime, their ho-hum lives will be ruled by ineffective bodies.

And you? Well, my two patients, my two friends, my own struggles, and *you* are the reasons Jerry and I have written this book. I pray you will experience the multiple benefits of physical fitness, personal fulfillment, and spiritual growth. The road to wholeness starts today.

APPENDIX 1

CANADIAN PHYSICAL ACTIVITY READINESS QUESTIONNAIRE*

If any of the following questions are answered yes, physical activity might be inappropriate and medical advice should be sought regarding the type and intensity of exercise permissible.

_____ Has your doctor ever said you have heart trouble?

_____ Do you frequently suffer from pains in your heart or chest?

_____ Do you often feel faint or have episodes of severe dizziness?

_____ Has a doctor ever told you that you have a bone or joint problem such as arthritis that has been aggravated by exercise or might be made worse with exercise?

_____ Is there a good physical reason not mentioned above why you should not follow an activity program, even if you wanted to?

_____ Are you over age 69 and not accustomed to vigorous exercise?

Be warned: A "start low—go slow" approach to exercise should allow everyone to start. Very few of you are eligible to sneak off to the sidelines and become spectators.

*From the British Columbia Ministry of Health

148

APPENDIX 2

A 40-year-old man might want to follow this progression as he begins his program:

Frequency (times per week)	Duration (minutes)	Intensity	No. of weeks
3	15	moderate (60-65% of predicted maximum heart rate)	3-4
4	15	moderate	3-4
5	15	moderate	3-4
5	20	moderate	3-4
5	25	moderate	3-4
5	25	moderate (65-70% of predicted maximum heart rate, progressing to 85%)	3-4

The range of progression should slow with age. Some guidelines:

Age of subject	Increase every
30+	2-3 weeks
40+	3-4 weeks
50+	4-5 weeks
60+	5-6 weeks
70+	6-7 weeks

Some muscular soreness may be experienced after each increase. But this will be minimal to nonexistent if you are very careful.

APPENDIX 3

Activity	Caloric cost per minute	Time taken to burn approx. 200 calories
Calisthenics	5.0	40 minutes
Walking (3.5 mph)*	5.6	36 minutes
Cycling (10 mph)	8.5	24 minutes
Swimming (crawl)	9.0	22 minutes
Skipping rope (120/min.)	10.0	20 minutes
Jogging	10.0	20 minutes
Running	15.0	14 minutes

(This chart is taken from *Physiology of Fitness*, by Brian J. Sharkey.)

*One can increase the caloric expenditure of walking with "dynamic walking."

The calories burned for these activities will vary from person to person depending upon weight, terrain, weather factors, skill, and so on.

Here's how to burn those 2,000 weekly calories without strenuous sports or structured workouts.

Situation	Activity	Calories/weekly
On the job and at home	2 flights of stairs daily	300
Interoffice walking	1-2 miles daily	750
Leisure walking	1-2 hours or 5 miles per week	350
Moderate sports (golf, tennis, swimming)	2 hours per week	750
	TOTAL	2,150

(This chart is taken from *Rx Being Well*, July/August 1986.)

CALORIES USED PER MINUTE OF EXERCISE

Activity	Calories Burned per Minute	
	Wt.: 115-150 lb.	Wt.: 150-195 lb.
Aerobic dancing	6-7	8-9
Basketball	9-11	11-15
Bicycling	5-6	7-8
Golf	3-4	4-5
Jogging (5 mph)	9-10	12-13
Jogging (7 mph)	10-11	13-14
Rowing machine use	5-6	7-8
Sexual intercourse	4-5	5-6
Skiing (downhill)	8-9	10-12
Skiing (cross-country)	11-12	13-16
Swimming	5-6	7-10
Tennis (doubles)	5-7	7-8
Walking (2 mph)	2-3	3-4
Walking (4 mph)	4-5	6-7

NOTE: 3,500 calories burned = loss of 1 pound of body weight.

(The chart above is taken from *Rx Being Well*, July/August 1986.)

Appendix 4

The "Exercise Across America" Challenge*

The American Running and Fitness Association sells kits that provide you the various miles across each state and the total miles across the United States (2,775 miles). (Send $6.50 to the American Running and Fitness Association, 4405 East West Highway, No. 405, Bethesda, MD 20814.) *The kit provides not only actual miles but mile equivalencies.* For example, each of the following activity durations is the eqivalent of running one mile:

17 minutes of aerobic dance

12 minutes of basketball

23 minutes of calisthenics

20 minutes of golf

11 minutes of jump roping

9 minutes of karate

10 minutes of racquetball

12 minutes of rowing

16 minutes of downhill skiing

10 minutes of stair climbing

14 minutes of tennis

14 minutes of weight training

The easiest state to cross is Rhode Island (27 miles). The hardest state to cross is Alaska (858 miles), with Texas being the second hardest (661 miles).

*The information above is taken from the "Exercise Across America" kit, American Running and Fitness Association.

APPENDIX 5

WEIGHT-FOR-HEIGHT TABLE

SUGGESTED WEIGHTS FOR ADULTS

Height*	Weight in pounds**	
	19 to 34 years	*35 years and over*
5'0"	97-128	108-138
5'1"	101-132	111-143
5'2"	104-137	115-148
5'3"	107-141	119-152
5'4"	111-146	122-157
5'5"	114-150	126-162
5'6"	118-155	130-167
5'7"	121-160	134-172
5'8"	125-164	138-178
5'9"	129-169	142-183
5'10"	132-174	146-188
5'11"	136-179	151-194
6'0"	140-184	155-199
6'1"	144-189	159-205
6'2"	148-195	164-210
6'3"	152-200	168-216
6'4"	156-205	173-222
6'5"	160-211	177-228
6'6"	164-216	182-234

*Without shoes.
**Without clothes.

The higher weights in the ranges generally apply to men who tend to have more muscle and bone; the lower weights more often apply to women who have less muscle and bone.

Appendix 6

Body Mass Index (BMI)*

BMI = a person's weight in kilograms divided by height in meters squared. (BMI=kg/m^2).

In general, a person 35 or older is obese if he or she has a BMI of 27 or more. For people age 34 or younger, a BMI of 25 or more indicates obesity. A BMI of more than 30 usually is considered a sign of moderate to severe obesity.

BODY WEIGHTS IN POUNDS
ACCORDING TO HEIGHT AND BODY MASS INDEX[†]

	Body Mass Index (kg/m^2)													
	19	20	21	22	23	24	25	26	27	28	29	30	35	40
Height (in.)						Body weight (lb.)								
58	91	96	100	105	110	115	119	124	129	134	138	143	167	191
59	94	99	104	109	114	119	124	128	133	138	143	148	173	198
60	97	102	107	112	118	123	128	133	138	143	148	153	179	204
61	100	106	111	116	122	127	132	137	143	148	153	158	185	211
62	104	109	115	120	126	131	136	142	147	153	158	164	191	218
63	107	113	118	124	130	135	141	146	152	158	163	169	197	225
64	110	116	122	128	134	140	145	151	157	163	169	174	204	232
65	114	120	126	132	138	144	150	156	162	168	174	180	210	240
66	118	124	130	136	142	148	155	161	167	173	179	186	216	247
67	121	127	134	140	146	153	159	166	172	178	185	191	223	255
68	125	131	138	144	151	158	164	171	177	184	190	197	230	262
69	128	135	142	149	155	162	169	176	182	189	196	203	236	270
70	132	139	146	153	160	167	174	181	188	195	202	207	243	278
71	136	143	150	157	165	172	179	186	193	200	208	215	250	286
72	140	147	154	162	169	177	184	191	199	206	213	221	258	294
73	144	151	159	166	174	182	189	197	204	212	219	227	265	302
74	148	155	163	171	179	186	194	202	210	218	225	233	272	311
75	152	160	168	176	184	192	200	208	216	224	232	240	279	319
76	156	164	172	180	189	197	205	213	221	230	238	246	287	328

[†]Each entry gives the body weight in pounds for a person of a given height and body mass index. Pounds have been rounded off. **To use the table,** find the appropriate height in the left-hand column. Move across the row to a given weight. The number at the top of the column is the body mass index for the height and weight.

*Adapted from G. A. Bray and D. S. Gray, *Obesity: Part I*, 429-41.

What your BMI means:

20 to 25: You're doing something right. People in this group live the longest.

26 to 30: You're overweight and have an increased risk of developing high levels of blood cholesterol, blood pressure, blood glucose, and blood insulin.

Above 30: Consider yourself obese. That makes you more susceptible to diabetes, coronary heart disease, cancer, and diseases of the digestive tract.

Below 20: You're fine—if you're in good physical shape and if you aren't suffering from a disease—like cancer—that's causing you to be underweight.

WORKS CITED

Books

Baxter, Richard. *The Saints' Everlasting Rest*. New York: Revell, 1962.

Brand, Paul, and Phillip Yancey. *Pain: The Gift Nobody Wants*. New York: HarperCollins, 1988.

Bray, D. S. *Obesity*. Part I. Pathogenesis. West J. Med., 1988.

Buttrick, George A. *Devotional Classics*. Ed. Richard Foster and James Smith. San Francisco: HarperCollins, 1993.

Cooper, Kenneth. *The Aerobic Program for Total Well-Being*. New York: M. Evans and Company, 1982.

Covey, Stephen R. *The Seven Habits of Highly Effective People*. New York: Simon & Schuster, 1989.

Dossey, Larry. *Prayer Is Good Medicine*. New York: HarperCollins, 1996.

Foreyt, John P., and Ken Goodrick. *Living Without Dieting*. Houston: Harrison Publishing, 1992.

Frankl, Viktor E. *Man's Search for Meaning*. Boston: Beacon Press, 1984.

Girzone, Joseph P. *Never Alone*. New York: Double Day, 1994.

Lewis, C. S. *The Problem of Pain*. New York: Macmillan Publishing Co., 1945.

Lodahl, Michael. *The Story of God*. Kansas City: Beacon Hill Press of Kansas City, 1994.

Lyons, George. *Holiness in Everyday Life*. Kansas City: Beacon Hill Press of Kansas City, 1992.

Magnusson, Anna. *The Village: A History of Quarrier's*. Glasgow: Quarrier's Homes, 1984.

Merton, Thomas. *Devotional Classics*. Ed. Richard J. Foster and James Smith. San Francisco: HarperCollins, 1993.

———. *The Wisdom of the Desert*. Boston: Shambhala, 1994.

Minirth, Frank, and Paul Meier. *Happiness Is a Choice*. Grand Rapids: Baker Book House, 1978.

Muggeridge, Malcolm. *Something Beautiful for God*. New York: Image Books, 1977.

Muller, Wayne. *Legacy of the Heart: The Spiritual Advantages of a Painful Childhood*. New York: Simon and Schuster, 1992.

Myers, David, Ph.D. *The Pursuit of Happiness*. New York: Evon, 1993.

Nieman, David C. *The Sports Medicine Fitness Course*. Palo Alto, Calif.: Bull Publishing Co., 1986.

Peck, M. Scott, M.D. *In Search of Stones: A Pilgrimage of Faith, Reason, and Discovery*. New York: Hyperion, 1995.

Purkiser, W. T. *When You Get to the End of Yourself*. Kansas City: Beacon Hill Press of Kansas City, 1970.

Seligman, Martin E. P. *Learned Optimism*. New York: A. A. Knopf, 1991.

Sharkey, Brian J. *Physiology of Fitness*. Champaign, Ill.: Human Kinetics Publishers, 1984.

Sheehan, George. *Personal Best*. Emmaus, Pa.: Rodale Press, 1989.

Tozer, Aiden Wilson. *The Knowledge of the Holy*. San Francisco: Harper and Row Publishers, 1961.

Wynkoop, Mildred Bangs. *Foundations of Wesleyan-Arminian Theology*. Kansas City: Beacon Hill Press of Kansas City, 1967.

ARTICLES

Bernstein, L. and R. K. Ross. "Physical Exercise and Reduced Risk of Breast Cancer in Young Women." *Journal of National Cancer Institute*, vol. 86, No. 18 (September 21, 1994).

Byrd, Randolph, M.D. *Journal of Christian Nursing*, vol. 12, No. 1.

Christensen, Michael J. "Mirror of Christ: Francis the Saint." *One*, May/June 1983, 10-13.

Clark, Nancy. "Nutrition Knowledge, Answers to the Top Ten Questions." *The Physician and Sports Medicine*, vol. 24, No. 10 (October 1996).

Cohen, J., M.D. "The Meeting of Chronic Pain Challenge." *Psychobiology of Pain*. American Pain Society, January 1995.

"Dump the Diet." *Runners World*, January 1997.

Ebron, Angela. "Why Goofing Off Is Good for You." *Family Circle*, February 1, 1996, 28.

Gasque, W. Ward. "Is Man's Purpose an Enigma?" *Christianity Today*, July 29, 1977.

Greenfield, Meg. "Don't Believe All the Epitaphs." *Newsweek*, November 16, 1987.

Johns Hopkins Medical Letter, *Health After 50*, July 1996.

Johns Hopkins Medical Letter, *Health After 50*, April 1997.

"Improved Respiratory Muscle Endurance of Highly Trained Cyclists." *International Journal of Sports Medicine* 12 (1991): 26.

Kerr, Laurette. "Good Grief, Where Are the Perfect People?" *Diabetes Forecast*, January 1994.

McCullough, Michael E. "Prayer and Health: Conceptual Issues, Research Review, and Research Agenda." *Journal of Psychology and Theology* 23, No. 1 (1995): 15-19.

Larson, David B. National Institute of Health Care Research. Rockville, MD.

O'Connor, Gerald T. "Physical Exercise and Reduced Risk of Nonfatal Myocardial Infarction." *American Journal of Epidemiology.* Johns Hopkins University School of Hygiene and Public Health 28, No. 9 (November 1994): 4.

Olsson, Karl. "The Bad Samaritan." *Faith at Work,* June 1973.

Ornish, Dean. "Can Lifestyle Changes Reverse Coronary Arteriosclerosis?" *Hospital Practice,* May 15, 1991.

Peterson, D. I. "Smoking and Pulmonary Function." *Archives of Environmental Health,* February 1968.

The President's Council on Physical Fitness and Sports, 1971.

Report of the Surgeon General, *Physical Activity & Fitness Research Digest,* series 2, No. 6 (July 1996).

Report of the Surgeon General. *Physical Activity and Health.* Washington, D.C.: At-A-Glance, 1996.

Rx Being Well, July / August 1986.

Taylor, Paul. "Who Has Time to Be a Family?" *Washington Post Weekly,* January 14-20, 1991.

Thomas, Gary. "Doctors Whom Pray: How the Medical Community Is Discovering the Power of Prayer." *Christianity Today,* January 6, 1997.

Wellness Health Letter, September 1995.

Wulff, Joan. "How's Your Friend Life?" *HIS,* October 1981.

The Writing Group for the DISC Collaborative Research Group. "Efficacy and Safety of Lowering Dietary Intake of Fat and Cholesterol." *Journal of the American Medical Association,* vol. 273, No. 18 (May 10, 1995).

Yaconelli, Mike. "Billiard Ball Relationships." *The Wittenburg Door,* April / May 1980.

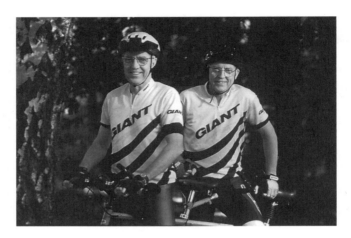

JERRY HULL is the chairman of the Department of Social Work and Sociology at Northwest Nazarene College, as well as an ordained minister. He and his wife, Barbara, live in Nampa, Idaho.

LARRY HULL is a founder and practicing physician at the Washington Orthopedic Center. He resides in Centralia, Washington, with his wife, Aarlie.